The Very Essence

The
Very Essence

Lisa Burke

Philip Chambers
(ITEC Dip)

Simon Mallinson
(IIHT Dip, IIHT Massage Dip)

Second edition

Likisma Presentations Limited

Always consult your doctor if in any doubt about your health. If taking medication or treatment from a medical or other complementary practitioner you should seek their advice before using Essential Oils as part of a home treatment.

Aromatherapy is a complementary therapy and should not replace any existing medication you have been prescribed.

Please follow the guidelines for the use of Essential Oils detailed in this book and read the information contained in Chapter 10 'General precautions' carefully.

The authors and publisher do not accept responsibility for any problems or any adverse reaction caused by the inappropriate use of oils, the use of poor quality oils or oils that have been stored incorrectly.

First published in August 1996 by
Likisma Presentations Limited
Dolphin House, Denington Road,
Wellingborough, Northants
NN8 2QH

Reprinted May 1997
Reprinted November 1997
Reprinted May 1998
Reprinted November 1998
Reprinted May 1999
Second edition December 1999
Reprinted June 2000
Third edition September 2002
Reprinted March 2004
Reprinted November 2005

British Library Cataloguing in Publication Data

A catalogue record for this book is available from the British Library.

ISBN 0 9528429 3 9

Printed and bound in Great Britain by
Cox & Wyman Ltd, Reading, Berkshire

Contents

Acknowledgements

O ur first thanks must go to our partners and families. They have had to suffer a great deal through the production of this book, and have all remained supportive and sane!

Our next thanks must go to all those Aromatherapists, writers, organisations, etc, who have informed us and many millions of others about the benefits and joys of Aromatherapy. Their work, research, writings and practice have been a great source of material for this book.

We must pay tribute to the man who began the modern revival in the therapeutic use of Essential Oils, Professor Renee Gattefosse. Without him we may never have discovered this wonderful world of healing aromas.

Chapter 1

Introduction

There are many books now available on Aromatherapy (see 'Further reading' at the end of the book for just a few of these titles). Why then do we need another? *The Very Essence* is, we believe, just that - the essential information you need in order to use and enjoy essences and Aromatherapy. We have felt for some time that with all the books currently available there is usually something of which we would have liked to have seen more or less in each book. Some are too detailed on methods; others do not include all appropriate oils; not all include an easy-to-use reference section on conditions and their treatment, and so on.

In this book, therefore, we have tried to present you with all the essential information on Aromatherapy and how to benefit from its use without over-loading you with facts, figures and opinions. We think that we have succeeded in this effort and hope that you enjoy reading this book and using it as an easy reference when you begin to use Essential Oils - as we are sure you will do!

Over the past 20 to 30 years complementary therapies in general and Aromatherapy in particular have become very well known and extensively used both by professionals and amateurs at home all over the world. It is very fashionable, but, as with all complementary therapies, it is no new trend.

There are many prescribed and over-the-counter medicines today that owe their existence to the plant world; for example aspirin, which was derived from the willow tree, Friar's Balsam, an inhalation derived from Benzoin Essential Oil, and so on. Plants have always been a source of healing since man first walked upright, and if we take care of our amazing natural resource they may yet provide the answers to all our ailments.

Put simply, Aromatherapy is the use of Essential Oils that have been extracted from raw organic material for therapeutic purposes.

Essential Oils are very volatile substances that are very complex chemical compounds. They are the vital elements of all plants, and can contain over 100 different chemical elements.

Most people will associate Aromatherapy with fragrances and the perfume industry. Aroma is, of course, a large part of Aromatherapy, but it is much more than just a nice smell. Essential Oils are used to provide remedies to many common ailments and are very powerful alternatives to many laboratory-produced medicines and cleansers (Tea Tree, for example, is about 12 times stronger than carbolic acid in its antiseptic, antiviral and antifungal properties, but it is still gentle and non-irritant).

The oils are extracted from various parts of various plants and are soluble in alcohol, ether and other oils. There are many different colours from clear to green and their consistency ranges from water-like to thick and heavy. They are produced in many parts of the world, and the same species of plant grown in different countries under different soil, altitude and climate conditions will produce oils that differ in their chemical make-up and therefore therapeutic properties. Country of origin is therefore very important.

Some oils are fairly easy to obtain because they are easily extracted (for example citrus oils squeezed from the rind), or the plant may be very rich in oil (for example Lavender). Other oils are very difficult to obtain - it takes 60,000 rose blossoms to make one ounce of rose oil. These differences are reflected in the prices of oils. All true Essential Oils are expensive to produce because they are so labour-intensive. Mechanised harvesting will often destroy the parts of the plants from which the oil is to be obtained.

There are many different ways of using Essential Oils, from neat to massage, and these are all explained in more detail in Chapter 2, 'Methods of use'. In short, any method of safely introducing the oils into the body will be beneficial, but there are some precautions you need to take; please therefore read Chapter 10 on general precautions before you start to use Essential Oils. Though most Essential Oils are generally regarded as safe, they are chemicals that affect the body and should be treated with respect and used correctly.

A brief history of Aromatherapy

Some of the earliest writings on the use of aromatic or Essential Oils on the body have been found in China, dating from some 2000 years BC. Several oils are referred to and their properties are basically the same as they are today. Most evidence of widespread use of oils comes from ancient Egypt where the 'doctors' of the time (who were also the priests) used oils in their offerings to their gods; it is well known that oils were extensively used in preserving and embalming the dead there.

In India in 2000 BC various writings mention 'perfumers and incense-sellers'. The evidence suggests that oils were used mainly for their aroma and this is possibly the case. However, when we get to the fourth century BC we find Hippocrates, who is acknowledged as the father of medicine, writing that 'the way to health is to have an aromatic bath and scented massage every day'. Here we have a clear link being made between aroma and health, as well as massage and health.

There are many other writings throughout ancient history in many civilisations on the use of Essential Oils. Another famous name is the more recent tenth-century Arabian physician Avicenna, who wrote many books on the properties and benefits of Essential Oils. In the 13th century, largely as a result of the Crusades, a growing industry in perfume-making developed in France, which formed the basis of that country's continued reputation as the home of perfumery. Between roughly 1200 and 1600 there were many books on and practitioners in herbal medicine throughout Europe. In the 17th century Lavender gained a well-deserved reputation as a preventative to the plague and was used extensively in posies, perfumed gloves and in other ways.

The popularity and benefits of Essential Oils continued to develop right through to the early 19th century, with Lavender leading the way. During that century the 'age of science' began to assume the lead position with its new, synthetic and very powerful substances. These were very effective, by and large, but were usually accompanied by many and various side-effects. The use of Essential Oils as therapy began to lose ground and over a short period of time they reverted to their other role as perfumes.

The resurgence of interest in Essential Oils for therapy can be attributed to two major events; the move during the present century towards purer, more natural forms of treatment, and the work of Professor Renee Gattefosse in France. Gattefosse was a chemist who began working with Essential Oils in the First World War by using principally Chamomile, Lavender and Lemon on wounded French soldiers. The famous Gattefosse story is that he first discovered the healing power of Lavender while experimenting in his laboratory. He burned his hand and plunged it into the nearest bowl, which actually contained Lavender oil. He was amazed at the rapid recovery of the burn and the lack of any blisters or scars. It is interesting to note that the healing power of oils, particularly Lavender, which had been well known only 100 years before this, had been so completely lost that it had to be rediscovered.

Gattefosse actually coined the term 'aromatherapie' to describe the use of Essential Oils for therapeutic purposes. His work was continued by another French physician, Dr Jean Valnet, who also wrote a book called *Aromatherapie*. Another biochemist, Marguerite Maury, translated the work of Gattefosse and Valnet into formulas and recipes, which her physician husband then used with his patients and their work produced a great deal of empirical evidence about the use and benefits of Essential Oils. Marguerite Maury spent a great deal of her time in Great Britain teaching a whole new generation of Aromatherapists like Daniele Ryman, who continue the work to this day.

The renewed interest in all alternative therapies over the past few years is part of a general move towards purer, more natural forms of treatment and a rejection of the 'popping a pill for a quick cure' mentality that became predominant in the middle 1900s. Many people are also more aware of their own bodies and health issues in general, and are more informed about the effects and side-effects of orthodox medication.

It is to be hoped that in time alternative therapies will become part of a comprehensive approach to health care, and practitioners in these fields will be as recognised as all other medical practitioners. This is beginning to happen with some GPs providing some of these services in their centres or referring patients to reputable therapists.

None of the above should be seen as devaluing the very great benefit that conventional medicine can provide for many conditions. Complementary means exactly that; to be used in conjunction with conventional medicine and with the knowledge of your doctor when receiving his or her treatment. Always consult your doctor if there is any possibility that you may have a serious condition needing treatment.

Quality of oils

The quality and purity of Essential Oils is of vital importance. Unless the oil is of top quality and extracted by one of the approved methods, it is of no use therapeutically even if the aroma is exact. Until recently Essential Oils have been largely produced for the perfume industry and the amounts needed meant that many were produced in the laboratory in order to ensure uniformity. There is, therefore, a lot of these types of oils on the market. Some blended oils, ie a base oil with Essential Oils already added, can sometimes be misleadingly labelled as 'pure Essential Oils'.

One of the other dangers with Essential Oils is that some of the more expensive examples can easily be adulterated with cheaper oils to make them go further. Sandalwood, for example, can be diluted with castor without easy detection; Juniperberry can be adulterated with turpentine; Neroli often has Petitgrain added; and Rose is stretched by adding Geranium and Palmarosa.

Oils can be synthesised in the laboratory to produce an exact aroma. These will tend to be cheaper as they are easier to produce, but they will not be as effective since some of the trace elements in Essential Oils are still unknown to us, so they cannot be perfectly duplicated artificially.

Always buy your oils from a reputable, reliable source. Check that the oil is the correct one, ie the Latin name should be evident somewhere.

Storing oils

Essential Oils are very volatile, ie they evaporate quickly when exposed to the air. Air will also cause oxidisation of oils, and they are also affected by light and heat. Always buy and store your

Essential Oils in dark glass bottles with air-tight, child-proof caps. Keep them in a cool dark place; the fridge is suitable if it is kept at a reasonable temperature (some oils may turn cloudy or thicken if kept too cold).

A bottle of Essential Oil, if stored correctly, can last and maintain its quality for at least 12 months. Some, like Patchouli, actually mature and mellow with age, and there is a market for these 'old masters'. Once blended with other oils, and in carriers, oils will begin to oxidise, weaken and go rancid. This process, however, does take three months or more, and if you store your blends under the same conditions as your Essential Oils they should be perfectly satisfactory if used within the three months.

How oils are obtained

There are several different methods of extracting the oil from the raw material. The two most often used are distillation and expression.

Distillation
The most widely used method of producing Essential Oils is by steam distillation. A quantity of the plant is added to a large still, covered with water and steamed. The resulting vapour is put through a condenser, which cools the steam and reduces it back to water, collected in a large container with oil floating on the top, or lying on the bottom if it is heavier than the water. It is then simply a matter of carefully separating the oil from the water.

Expression
Citrus oils are extracted by this method, which is probably one of the easiest to do yourself. Commercially this process is performed today by machine, but it is perfectly possible to do it by hand or with a small press. The peel of the fruit is squeezed on to a sponge, and when the sponge is saturated the oil can be squeezed out of it. It is as simple as that.

Other methods of extraction
Three other extraction methods are sometimes used for particular oils. **Enfleurage** and **Maceration** are based on the fact that fat

absorbs Essential Oils. Briefly, flowers are laid on cold fat and changed regularly until the fat is saturated with oil (Enfleurage), or bunches of flowers are dipped repeatedly in hot fat until it is saturated (Maceration). In both cases the resultant block of fat (called a 'pomade') is washed in alcohol, which is then evaporated to release the oils.

Solvent extraction, although not favoured by us, is increasingly being used as it is easier and cheaper than the above methods. Oil is absorbed by a heated solvent, for example petroleum. After filtering, the solvent (now called a 'concrete') is treated as a pomade, as in Enfleurage or Maceration.

How oils work

In order for Essential Oils to have any effect they need to be absorbed by the body. There are only two acceptable and safe ways of doing this, Inhalation and Absorption.

Inhalation

Can you think of a smell that stimulates you in some way? The smell of freshly baked bread, for example. What pictures does it conjure up? How does it make you feel? The fact that you could answer these questions demonstrates just how powerful an aroma can be. Why have supermarkets all recently begun to bake their own bread on the premises? Mainly because the smell of baking bread stimulates people into feeling good and possibly hungry.

Aromas work by stimulating the olfactory nerves at the back of the nose, which then send messages to the olfactory bulb situated in the third ventricle area of the brain - the limbic system. This part of the brain is responsible for our primitive drives of sex, hunger and thirst. The pituitary gland and hypothalamus are both also situated in this area, and these organs are responsible for the release of hormones into the circulation system that control many body functions and release emotions and memories. Stimulating the olfactory nerves can therefore have a direct effect on the body.

The pituitary gland is the leader of the endocrine system and plays a part in regulating the production of hormones by all the glands:

- Lachrymal - the gland that produces tears, which help to lubricate the eye and wash away foreign bodies.

- Salivary - the gland that produces saliva, helping to lubricate the mouth and begin the digestive process.

- Thyroid - the gland responsible for the development of sex organs, and which also produces T-lymphocytes, an important part of the body's immune system.

- Parathyroid - these four glands maintain the balance of calcium and phosphorus in the blood and bone.

- Adrenal - these glands lie over both kidneys and control sodium and potassium, stimulate the storage of glucose and affect the production of sex hormones. Adrenaline is also produced, which is a powerful vasoconstrictor, raising blood pressure and blood sugar and activated by strong emotions like excitement, fear, anger, and so on.

- Gonads - in men these are the testes, in women the ovaries. They produce the sex hormones oestrogen, progesterone and testosterone, which are responsible for the development of breasts, pubic and axillary hair, voice changes, muscle mass, etc.

- Pancreas - a part of the pancreas produces insulin, which regulates the sugar level in the blood and the conversion of sugar into heat and energy.

- Pituitary - these glands secrete many hormones including the growth-promoting hormone; hormones for male and female gonad activity; hormones to regulate the thyroid; and others to regulate the adrenal gland. Other hormones produced control uterine muscles, mammary glands and kidneys.

The hypothalamus is part of the neurological system, which influences the autonomic nervous system, ie the part of the nervous system that controls all the involuntary muscles, such as the heart, lungs, etc. It also works with the pituitary gland in regulating female sex hormones, and is connected to the control of appetite.

As you can see, the inhalation of Essential Oils can have a powerful effect on the hormones produced in the endocrine system. Essential Oils that are useful for hormonal conditions would therefore probably be most effective if inhaled.

Absorption

Essential Oils are absorbed into the skin and from there directly to the blood stream. There are several methods that achieve this, including bath, compress, massage, neat, etc. Inhaling oils will also achieve absorption via the lungs, from where they enter the bloodstream in the surrounding blood vessels.

Essential Oils appear to work in the body in two ways. The chemicals in the oils find their way directly into the bloodstream and increase or boost the levels of vitamins, minerals, proteins, acids and so on that are naturally produced in the body. They seek out the particular parts of the body that are deficient in some way and provide a supplementary addition to the chemical balance in the body.

The other way oils seem to work is that they trigger the body's own immune system by locking on to particular molecules in the body and sending a signal to the immune system to produce T-cells and B-cells, which are both responsible for attacking and killing invading organisms.

However it works, osmosis is a very effective way of introducing Essential Oils to the body and rapidly dispersing them to the required areas.

The absorption rate of Essential Oils varies between individuals and oils. Penetration through the skin takes only a few minutes in all people, even if the skin is congested, but absorption into the bloodstream and from there to the appropriate organs will vary, depending on the subject's size, circulation and general health, from between 70 minutes and six hours.

The oil is expelled from the body through urine, faeces, perspiration and exhalation, and the rate will again vary between individuals from between three to 14 hours. It is thought that Essential Oils leave no toxins behind when expelled, unlike laboratory-produced medication, which can stay in the body for a very long time.

Empirical and scientific evidence of the effectiveness of Essential Oils and how they work is constantly being updated as more and more research into this art is undertaken. Aromatherapy is not a 'quack' remedy or a matter of belief - it works!

Chapter 2

Methods of use

*T*here are many ways of using Essential Oils, and at least one of them will be right for you. Many people are 'turned off' Aromatherapy because they think, or have been told, that it's messy or fiddly and takes a lot of time. How much easier it is to pop a pill into the mouth, or spread some handy ointment on the body!

Yet how much nicer to put a few drops of Lavender in a room burner and allow the lovely aroma to permeate the whole house while it is quietly and efficiently, without side-effects, relieving that headache!

Aromatherapy is easy, very pleasant to use, and fun; it fits into our modern way of life quite well. Unfortunately most people still think of Aromatherapy as a branch of massage, and that massage is complicated, difficult and time-consuming. Yes, it is one of the best ways of using Essential Oils, but there are so many other ways that can be just as effective.

Many of these methods are described here. It is not an exhaustive list and you may well know, or you may discover, other methods. **However, we strongly advise against taking oils internally.**

Room burner (oil burner; diffuser; vaporiser)
Room burners are specifically made for use with Essential Oils. You can now buy them at many different retail outlets in different shapes, sizes, designs and patterns. There are some points you should check before buying: make sure that the bowl element of the burner is fairly deep; that the candle chamber is fairly large and has sufficient holes to allow excess heat to escape; and that the base of the burner is fairly thick, or has a raised rim to lift the centre of the base from the surface on which you are placing it. Also remember that a glazed burner will not crack, burn or stain, and is easy to keep clean. Night candles can be used in a burner, but do use candles that have a liquid wax and a

good quality wick so that it will not smell when alight or smoke when blown out (check the packet for suitability).

How to use: Place a small amount of cold water in the bowl, enough to fill it but leaving some space for water expansion. The Essential Oils of your choice are then dropped into the water (between 3 and 5 drops will normally be used depending on the size of the bowl and the amount of water being used). Place the candle in the chamber, light it and leave in a safe place. Use for 20-25 minutes (this will, of course, depend on the size of the room/house, the flow of air via opening and closing doors, the passage of people through the room, the type of oil used, etc).

Benefits: Psychological conditions can be treated very effectively with a room burner. Headaches respond well to this method and all respiratory problems can be treated in this way. A major use of the room burner is to create a 'therapeutic atmosphere' in a room where someone is ill. Using the room burner is an ideal alternative to environmentally unfriendly commercial room fresheners to fragrance your home. The room burner is also a good preventative against airborne viruses and bacteria.

Bath

Using Essential Oils in the bath is one of the most enjoyable and effective methods in Aromatherapy. It is quick, easy and very pleasant. Most people still have baths in their homes, though there is an increasing trend towards having shower rooms/cubicles only. Be careful to clean the bath thoroughly after use if your bath has a plastic surface as Essential Oils may, over a long period of time, discolour or damage it.

How to use: Fill the bath, add the Essential Oil(s) (up to 6 drops or as directed), then agitate the water to disperse the oil. Soak in the bath for at least 10 minutes, and make sure the bathroom door is closed so that you get the benefit of inhaling the aroma as well as getting the oil directly into the body via the water. For some conditions, or if preferred, the Essential Oils can be diluted in a massage carrier oil first, which will help to disperse the oil throughout the water. Alternatively, a better solution would be to add approximately 10 ml of specially formulated fragrance-free bath carrier before adding the Essential Oils, which has the added benefits of moisturising the body, giving a bubble/foam bath and helping to carry the Essential Oil out of the bath. Do not use a fragranced bubble/foam bath as the chemicals they contain may interact with the chemicals in the Essential Oils.

Benefits: The use of oils in a bath is useful for all conditions but will be particularly beneficial for muscular and skin conditions, while respiratory problems will benefit from the inhalation of the aroma. Stress, anxiety and other mental health problems will also be improved. Sexual problems, such as impotence and frigidity, respond well to this treatment. Anyone suffering with insomnia will find a pre-retiring bath with Bergamot, Lavender, Neroli, Petitgrain or several other oils a great aid to a good restful sleep.

Lotions and creams
Essential Oils can be added to fragrance-free lotions or creams, but make sure that you use a very good quality product that is preferably lanolin-free (some people are sensitive to lanolin, which can cause a rash or itching).

How to use: Add the Essential Oil(s) to a jar/pot that has been very well cleaned. It should preferably be a dark glass jar to help preserve the oil and prevent it from reacting with a plastic bottle. The recommended dosage is from 1 to 2 drops for every 5 ml of lotion or 5 g of cream (see Chapter 4 for the exact quantity).

Apply lotion to the skin and rub until completely absorbed; this should only take a few seconds.

Cream should be applied to the skin and gently rubbed in. Leave the rest to sit on the surface of the skin and gradually release the oil into the body and the aroma into the nose.

Benefits: This is a particularly good way of treating most skin conditions such as eczema, psoriasis, which will benefit greatly. However, lotions and creams may make fungal conditions worse, so use with care for these. A lotion is an excellent way to get Essential

Oils rapidly into the bloodstream and is therefore useful for treating conditions such as circulation problems. Lotions and creams can be effectively used for headaches, while creams are a good way of treating respiratory conditions. Both are an essential medium for general body and skin care.

Inhalation

This is an old-fashioned remedy that has unfortunately been somewhat neglected in recent times due to the ascendency of pharmacological preparations such as cough mixtures, expectorants and so on. This is a very powerful method of use and should be preferred much more often.

How to use: Pour about a pint of very hot water into a bowl, then add up to 3 drops of Essential Oil(s) to the water; there is no need to agitate the water to disperse the oil. Cover your head with a towel and lean over the bowl, keeping your head about 9 or 10 inches above the bowl. Keep your eyes closed as the vapour will sting them. Breathe in for about 2 minutes, then lean back and relax for a couple of minutes. Repeat the treatment for up to a maximum of 10 minutes.

Benefits: Respiratory conditions will obviously benefit most from this treatment method. Eucalyptus, Niaouli, Scots Pine and several other oils are excellent decongestants renowned for their ability to help most respiratory conditions. Inhalation is also a good way of treating facial skin problems as its effect is the same as that achieved by a facial sauna. Asthmatics should not use this method as the concentration of aroma and steam may trigger an attack.

Compress

Compresses can be either hot or cold depending on the condition that is being treated. It is a well-known and frequently used treatment method for sports injuries in particular, though its uses are much wider than this and can be very effective for pain, swelling and inflammation.

How to use: The method is the same whether hot or cold. Add up to 5 drops of Essential Oil(s) to a basin or bowl of hot or icy cold water. Use a face-cloth, linen pad, cotton wool or other absorbent fabric and dip this into the water. Wring out the excess and place the pad on the affected area. Once the compress has achieved body temperature, renew it and continue as required. A hot compress can be held in place with crêpe bandage on joints or with cling-film on larger areas, for example the lower back.

Benefits: Most conditions characterised by 'aches', for example earache, backache, etc, should be treated with hot compresses, while sprains, fevers, inflammations and headaches should be treated with cold compresses. Sprains and varicose veins respond very well to the 'hot/cold' treatment, ie start with a cold compress then alternate between hot and cold compresses over the next few days, finishing with a cold one.

Massage
Giving and receiving a good massage is truly one of the most enjoyable experiences you can have. Many people say that they would love to have a massage but find it difficult to take the step and actually book one. Maybe it is the unfortunate association massage still has with other activities perpetuated by the media and stand-up comics! However, do overcome any inhibitions you have about massage as it is the best way of using Essential Oils. Its double therapeutic benefit is without equal and should be experienced by everyone.

You do not have to be a qualified masseur/se to be able to use this method for yourself, your partner or your family. Although it is difficult to learn massage from a book, you can gain some understanding of the techniques and movements. We are restricted for space here and will only cover back, face and neck, and abdominal massage. Trust your intuition and 'feel' your way, and you will soon find that you have a touch that transcends technique.

Contra-indications
Do not massage in the following conditions:

● Over areas of septic foci (spots, boils, etc)

● On contagious or infectious skin conditions

- Over the abdomen during pregnancy

- When there are cardio-vascular conditions

- Over areas of inflammation or pain

- On sprains, torn muscles and ligaments

- On burns

- Below or over an area of varicose veins

Preparation
Make sure that the room you are going to use is warm. Use soft lighting and relaxing music, if you wish, to enhance the mood. While giving and receiving a massage keep conversation to a minimum so that a quiet, relaxing atmosphere can be maintained.

Place a duvet, thick blankets, a sleeping bag or something similar on the floor and cover with a towel. Use two other towels to cover the parts of the body not being worked on so that the subject is kept warm. Make sure that you are not wearing any jewellery likely to catch on the person's skin, and also that your hands are in good condition, ie not chapped and rough, and with short, tidy fingernails.

Using oils
Prepare the oil you are going to use for the massage (see Chapter 4, 'Index of conditions'), and choose the carrier oil appropriate for the condition and skin type being treated (see 'Carrier oils' below). Use a maximum of 5 drops of Essential Oil to 10 ml of carrier.

Use a dark glass mixing bottle for your massage blend. After adding the Essential Oil(s) to the carrier agitate the mixing bottle very well to ensure that the oils are thoroughly blended. You may wish to use an aesthetically pleasing bowl in which to decant the blend for use in your massage.

If possible try to warm the oil to body temperature before use. Place a few drops of oil into the palm of your hand and rub your palms together to spread a thin layer over the whole of your hands.

The first mistake most people make is to apply too much oil, so follow the maxim 'the less the better'. Use just enough to give your hands a nice sheen - you should be able to hold your hands, fingertips pointing down, without oil dripping off. 7 or 8 ml of carrier oil should be enough to give a full body massage!

Massage movements

There are several different massage movements that all have their specific effect on the body. Two of the most useful ones are called Effleurage and Petrissage.

Effleurage is used to apply the oil evenly over the body, to warm and relax the area, to speed up the venous and lymph flow and allow the subject to get used to the masseur/se's touch. It should precede and succeed all other massage movements.

Effleurage is performed with the flat of the hand, with the fingers close together and, as far as is practical, the tips of the fingers turning upwards so that they avoid protuberances on the body. The hand should follow the contours of the body.

Effleurage movements are made towards the heart. They should be slow, rhythmic, and without breaks. Variation on the pressure applied should be made in the upward, or towards the heart, stroke.

Petrissage is normally applied with the balls of the thumb and/or fingers and is applied to soft tissue that has bone immediately beneath it. It is therefore suitable for use on any part of the body except the face (mild petrissage can be used on the jaw and temples) and abdomen. The balls of the digits are able to squeeze the soft tissue against the bone and so help to eliminate accumulated waste products from the muscles. It is important to use the ball of the digit - not the tip - and not to slide over the skin but to trap it securely so that a steady grinding movement can be achieved.

One other movement that can be used on the back and face is **Tapotement**. This is a fine, quick, 'drumming' vibratory movement, each finger being brought down in rapid succession on to the body - as if you were drumming your fingers impatiently on a desk. Use the balls of the fingers and apply an appropriate amount of pressure, deep on the back but light on the face. It is a good movement for small muscle areas, such as in the face, as it has a toning effect.

Back massage
Begin with the subject lying on his or her front, and kneel at their head facing down the body.

1   Use effleurage down the centre of the back, avoiding the spine, and when you are at the limit of your reach move your hands to the person's sides and bring your hands back up to the shoulders applying, light pressure as you go. Repeat the movement several times.

2   Use petrissage movements all the way around the edge of the shoulder blades with your fingers and thumbs. Apply to both shoulder blades at the same time.

3   Use petrissage movements across the shoulder blades.

4   Use petrissage movements between shoulder blades and spine up to the neck.

5   Move to the subject's side (whichever side is most comfortable for you), level with the hips and facing up the body, and use petrissage movements along the side of the person's spine from the base of the back up to the base of the neck using your thumbs.

6   Use tapotement all over the back at this point if you wish.

7   Effleurage up the back, from the base of the back, with the palms on either side of the spine applying light pressure. When you reach the shoulders move your hands over to just under the armpits and bring your hands down to the person's hips. Bring hands back together at the base of the spine. Repeat several times.

8   Move to the subject's side, level with the centre of the back and facing across the back. Place both your forearms on the centre of the back and, while applying quite a lot of pressure, move your arms apart until one arm is across the shoulders and the

other is across the hips. This is called 'stretching the back'. Return your hands to the centre of the back and place them palm down on the centre and rest there for a few seconds.

This completes a simple Aromatherapy back massage. Remember to keep your hands reasonably well oiled but don't over-use the oil. Try to keep your movements fluid and smooth; a jerky, heavy movement will disturb the subject and not achieve a relaxed state. Try to keep contact with the person, even when re-applying oil to your hands or moving to a new position.

Face and neck massage
This can either be performed with the subject on his or her back on the floor with you at the head, or with the subject sitting in a low, armless chair with you standing behind and the person's head resting on your tummy.

Make sure all the subject's jewellery, ie earrings, nasal rings, lip rings, etc, are removed. Oil your hands - use less oil than for the back - and use an appropriate carrier oil, for example Peach Kernel.

1   Begin on the neck. Place the palms of your hands on either side of the neck just above the collar bone with opposite fingers touching. Using light effleurage movements with both hands slowly bring them up to under the chin. Repeat three or four times. After the last movement, with your hands just under the chin, draw them apart towards the ears and continue up the sides of the face to the forehead.

2   Place the palms of your hands on each side of the subject's nose with the fingertips pointing down. Applying a very light pressure, move your hands down the face and, when you reach the chin, move them to the sides of the chin and bring them back up the sides of the face, then over to the start position again. Repeat once only.

3   Move your hands so that your thumbs are at the centre of the subject's forehead just below the hairline. Applying a light pressure, move your thumbs apart towards the sides of the head

twice. Move the thumbs down half an inch and repeat. Repeat the movement until the eyebrows have been massaged.

4   Perform the same movement over the eyelids, but reduce the pressure.

5   Move your thumbs to the bridge of the nose. Stroke down the nose from the bridge to the tip twice.

6   Move to the sides of the nose and repeat the movements as for the forehead until you reach the chin. Don't massage the lips.

7   From the centre of the chin, take the tissue between the thumbs and fingers of both hands and squeeze along the whole chin up to the jawbone.

8   At the jawbone use your fingers and petrissage the jaw joints gently.

9   Move your fingers to the subject's temples and gently petrissage.

10   Use tapotement all over face, being very careful to avoid the eyes.

11   Place your palms back in the original start position, making sure that the subject's eyes are covered by the heels of your hands. Applying a light pressure, move your hands over the cheeks towards the ears, stretching and smoothing the skin on the cheeks. When you reach the ears hold them with your thumbs in front and fingers behind, and gently stretch them away from the scalp. Squeeze along the ears with your thumbs and fingers from lobe to top.

12   Finish with a repeat of the first movement (effleurage) and end by stroking over the ears and coming off the back of the head.

13   Alternatively finish with a scalp massage. Start by 'combing out' the hair with your fingers. Continue with the same movements all over the scalp that you would use if you were

gently rubbing in shampoo to wash the hair. Finish by a repeat combing and coming off the back of the head.

Again remember to keep your movements smooth, fluid, rhythmic and fairly slow. This should be a relaxing, pleasant experience for you and the subject, so don't make them anxious or jumpy by being rough and jerky.

Abdominal massage

The subject should be laying on his or her back with arms by their sides. Remember that the abdomen is a delicate area with no protecting skeleton. The muscles covering the abdomen are, however, fairly strong, thick and elastic, which affords sufficient protection to the sensitive organs in that part of the body. All massage movements over the abdomen should be performed in a clockwise direction, as this follows the direction of the colon, one of the major organs in the abdomen.

1   Place yourself at the subject's side, next to the abdomen, facing across the body towards the subject's opposite foot. Choose whichever side is most comfortable for you - most people find the person's left side is best.

2   Using the palms of the hands, gently effleurage the abdomen by circling over it with both hands. As your hands cross keep contact with one hand while the other is moved over. Repeat the movement several times.

3   Using one hand only (your right if you are on the person's left or your left if on the person's right), begin to apply more pressure with your movement.

4   Move your hand in a circular movement over the groin, where pressure can be increased, then across to the opposite hip and pull up over the hip and side; then gently trace along the bottom of the rib cage. Half-way across smoothly turn your hand around so that your fingertips are facing towards you. Continue the movement under the ribs to the side of the subject

closest to you. Apply pressure along the side to the hip and push up over the hip, twisting your hand around as you go until your fingertips are pointing down towards the person's feet, and continue the movement over the groin. Repeat the whole movement three or four times.

5   Finish the massage by returning to the effleurage movement with which you began over the whole abdomen.

Benefits
There are many benefits to using massage. It is probably the best method to use for all psychological/emotional problems as the touch of another person on the body is healing in itself. Combined with the power of Essential Oils this is an unbeatable remedy. Obviously all muscular/skeletal conditions will benefit from massage, but do be careful if they are inflamed and painful or if being treated for a sprain. Toxin elimination is achieved very well by the use of massage, and cellulite in particular can be treated in this way. Massage increases the flow of lymph, which is responsible for manufacturing and distributing infection-fighting white blood cells - lymphocytes - throughout the body, and therefore will help to treat most infections and generally improve the immune system.

Neat
There are a few oils that are safe to use neat, ie without blending them first in a carrier of some sort. There is not total agreement about this in the Aromatherapy world, but there is a broad consensus that Chamomile, Lavender, Lemon and Tea Tree can all be used neat on the skin, and we recommend such use. There is no great therapeutic advantage in using other oils neat, apart from the fact that it is convenient and easy, so always blend other oils in a carrier. Always test the oils on your skin first if it is sensitive or if you have reacted to oils, perfumes, bath foams, etc, in the past. If you have a reaction after using an oil neat, see Chapter 10, 'General precautions'.

How to use: Simply apply the oil(s) neat from the bottle with the fingers or cotton wool/pads. Use only 1 or 2 drops for whatever complaint you are treating.

Benefits: The main benefit will be for skin problems: cuts, grazes, bites, stings, spots, boils, warts, verrucas and minor burns. Nosebleeds can also be relieved by using Lemon neat on cotton wool (see Chapter 4, 'Index of conditions and recommended treatments').

Other methods

There are many other methods of using Essential Oils, which all have their place and may be suitable for you and your lifestyle. The following is a brief summary of some of them.

Room sprays

Make a home-made room spray using a sprayer that has been thoroughly cleaned, to provide your own favourite aromas to freshen your home. They can also be a great help in keeping a 'sick room' clear of infections. It is perfectly possible to make a room spray using a simple solution of cold water with added Essential Oils (stick to a 5 drops to 10 ml maximum). This will mean that every time you use it you will have to make sure you shake it vigorously to disperse the oils in the water. You can 'fix' the aroma and also help to disperse the oils equally in the water by using distilled water (boiled then cooled water) and adding 10 per cent alcohol (preferably vodka).

Radiators and humidifiers

Drops of oil can be placed in a saucer of water placed on top of a radiator, or on to a ball of damp cotton wool placed behind the radiator. Drops of oil can also be added to the water in a humidifier.

All these methods can be used as an alternative to a room burner, but are not as effective and are a second best choice.

Shower

There are several other methods of introducing Essential Oils into the body using water as the medium. For most people the next alternative to the bath will be the shower. Using Essential Oils in the shower is not as difficult as it might seem. Use a fragrance-free bath carrier or a specially prepared fragrance-free shower gel on a sponge or face-cloth. Wash yourself as normal using the gel/bath carrier to which you have added 4 or 5 drops of Essential Oil(s), then rub the sponge/face-cloth over your body while continuing to stand under the running water.

Foot bath
For foot problems, and as a way of introducing Essential Oils into the body for other problems, a foot bath can be used. This can either be a piece of equipment specially made for the purpose or a bowl of warm water. Add 2-4 drops of oil to the bath, disperse and immerse feet for up to 20 minutes; adding a bath carrier will help. A hand bath can achieve the same result for hand problems, and is achieved in the same way, but only immerse for 10 minutes.

Tissue/handkerchief/pillow
Any method that allows inhalation of the oils is an alternative to steam inhalation. Some specific methods not mentioned so far are a tissue/handkerchief - add 1 or 2 drops of oil and sniff as required - and a pillow - place 1 or 2 drops of oil on to your pillow at night so that the oil can be inhaled throughout the night.

Pot-pourri
Although not a recognised therapeutic method, a pot-pourri is a pleasant way of creating an aromatic atmosphere in a house or sick room. Adding Essential Oils to a pot-pourri will fragrance a room and introduce the Essential Oils into the body through inhalation. Use a base note oil, or alcohol, to 'fix' the aroma in the pot-pourri.

Carrier oils

Essential Oils are concentrated and powerful and most cannot be used directly on the skin or they will cause irritation. Because of their concentration they need to be diluted in what are called 'carriers'. When used in a room burner, bath, foot bath, compress, room spray, etc, the carrier is water; lotions and creams are also carriers. The methods of use above explain these uses in more detail.

Alcohol can be used as part of a water-based carrier, as the Essential Oils will dissolve very easily in it; this is why many perfumes are alcohol-based. Of course perfume manufacturers will use particular grades of alcohol like ethanol, not the sort of alcohol that you would wish to drink! Buying perfume-grade alcohol is not easy and you will usually need a licence. A very good alternative is high-proof vodka; used as a 10% blend with water (distilled, or boiled then cooled, water is best), vodka will dissolve and disperse Essential Oils and also 'fix' an aroma.

Massage carrier oils

For massage with Essential Oils we recommend that you use a carrier oil made specifically for that use. These are all extracted by cold-pressing, ie they are put under high pressure in their natural, raw state when first harvested to squeeze out the oil, and neither heat nor steam is used in the process. This retains the nutrients in the oils (the proteins, minerals, vitamins, etc) that allow them to be readily absorbed by the skin.

Virtually any vegetable oil can be used as a carrier, but anything other than a specific massage carrier will have several drawbacks. All will be too heavy to be easily absorbed by the skin, and most are not cold-pressed and will often contain additives, flavourings or colouring. Ordinary vegetable oils have little or no therapeutic value in themselves, whereas massage carriers will have their own benefits.

Baby oils and other mineral oils are not suitable for Aromatherapy massage as they are specifically made to lie on the surface of the skin and will not be absorbed; however, they may be used if you want to massage without Essential Oils. They are still a second choice, though, as they will react to the friction of the massage and become tacky.

There are several different massage carrier oils produced, but we have detailed here the seven that are most often used.

SWEET ALMOND
Description: The oil is a clear pale yellow and is practically odourless. It contains vitamins, minerals, proteins and glucosides.
Uses: One of the most popular and useful of all carrier oils, Sweet Almond can be used for all skin types and is beneficial for most skin conditions. It can be used without adding other carrier oils. Avoid Bitter Almond oil.

PEACH KERNEL

Description: The oil is slightly paler than Sweet Almond but a little richer in texture. It contains vitamins and minerals.

Uses: It is good for all skins, particularly ageing, sensitive, inflamed and dry skin. It is particularly useful for facial massage. It can be used alone or with a few drops to Sweet Almond or Grapeseed added to enrich the blend.

EVENING PRIMROSE

Description: Again this is a pale yellow oil. It contains vitamins and minerals but its main constituent of benefit is gamma-linolenic acid (GLA), which is known to increase the body's production of hormones called prostaglandins.

Uses: It is very good for major skin conditions like psoriasis and eczema, is excellent for PMT and menopausal problems, and also used for arthritis and rheumatism. It is thought to be useful for multiple sclerosis and very helpful for heart disease as GLA controls cholesterol in the blood. Evening Primrose is often taken in capsule form and the oil is just as useful as a massage carrier or applied to the skin. It is powerful in its own right and should be used as part of a blend with another carrier, for example Peach Kernel; use as 10% only of the base.

GRAPESEED

Description: Again this is a very light coloured oil that is odourless. It contains vitamins, minerals and protein.

Uses: An all-purpose general carrier oil, it is useful for all skin types. It is absorbed very easily into the skin, and is used as a cleanser and toner. Most pre-prepared or shop-bought blends will have Grapeseed as a base because it has the least odour and is very light, allowing the aroma of the Essential Oil(s) to come through. Use Grapeseed on its own or as a blend.

JOJOBA

Description: This is actually a wax and therefore a unique carrier oil for use with Essential Oils. It has a yellow, golden colour and is thicker than most other carriers. It contains protein and minerals but its most useful quality is its consistency, which is very similar to natural collagen.

Uses: Due to its consistency Jojoba is usually accepted as the most useful massage carrier since it does not become sticky in use and is very rapidly absorbed into the skin. It is excellent for all skin types, is particularly good for haircare and is a favourite base for perfumes. Jojoba can be used on its own, but due to its luxuriousness we would recommend that you use it as 10-25% of a blend of carrier oils.

WHEATGERM
Description: This has a very strong orange colour and is very rich in vitamins E, A and B. The texture is very rich and thick, and it also has a stronger aroma than most carrier oils.
Uses: Wheatgerm has two major uses - it is excellent for regeneration of tissues and skin elasticity, making it the best oil to use for scar tissue and stretch marks, and it has powerful antioxidant qualities that can help to prevent degeneration and rancidity of any oil-based preparation. Add 10% of Wheatgerm to any blend to help preservation, and between 5% and 25% as part of a dry skin, tissue-regenerating or stretch-mark blend. This oil is not advised for use on its own as it is too heavy and has a noticeable aroma.

All oils, essential and carrier, have a limited 'shelf life' and over time will degenerate by oxidisation and become rancid. Adding Wheatgerm to any blend will extend its life, and a blend with Essential Oils will keep longer than the carrier alone. Follow the guidelines given under 'Storing oils' in Chapter 1.

Chapter 3

Blending oils

*B*lending Essential Oils is often referred to as the 'the art of Aromatherapy; the creative element'. It is also perhaps the most confusing and controversial aspect of Aromatherapy. Some Aromatherapists will say that there is no need and it is unnecessary to blend. At the other extreme some will promote the use of blends of five, six or more Essential Oils.

There are no rigid rules - it is largely a matter of taste and therapeutic value, but it is unlikely in our view that you will want or need to blend more than three oils together. However, it is quite possible to use more than three throughout a complete treatment for a particular condition, and it is also beneficial at times to use more than three in a range of different methods throughout an illness.

First of all, blending has to be separated into two different types - aesthetic and therapeutic.

Aesthetic blending

This is where several different oils may be blended together simply to achieve a particular aroma, as perfume manufacturers will do. In order to achieve a balanced blend of aromas, oils are classified in three different categories:

Top notes: An oil classified as a 'top note' is one that has the most immediate impact in a fragrance; this is the oil that gives the blend its distinctive first aroma. A top note will not last more than 24 hours before evaporating, and such oils tend to be sharp, penetrating, cold or hot oils, for example most citrus oils, Bergamot, Ginger, Tea Tree, etc. Top note oils are usually stimulating to mind and body.

Middle notes: Middle note oils are so described because they give a fragrance 'body'. They will have the aroma that comes through when the top note is beginning to evaporate and will smooth out the aroma and give it a warm, soft, mellow flavour. They last up to three days before evaporating and include Chamomile, Lavender, Rosemary, etc. Their main therapeutic benefits will tend to be for bodily functions.

Base notes: These oils will form the base of a blend and will tend to have deep, intense, heavy aromas. Some are not particularly pleasant when smelled from the bottle (Patchouli, for example), but when applied to the skin their aromas become much more pleasing. They are powerful aromas and should be used sparingly to avoid overpowering the blend. Oils in this category include Rose, Vetiver and Ylang Ylang. The aroma of some base note oils can last up to five days, and they also 'fix' an aroma, acting as a fragrance preservative allowing the aromas of the other oils to be effective for longer.

Some oils, because of their complex chemical composition, will be listed as both Top and Middle, or Middle and Base. These oils are very useful in a blend for 'bridging' between the notes and allowing the blend to have an overall character that moves smoothly from top to base.

The note given to each oil in our list of Essential Oils (Chapter 6) is a summary of several different Aromatherapists' views together with our own experience. These classifications should be used simply as a guide and we encourage you to experiment with aromas and find what oils and blends please you.

Blending proportions will again depend on taste, but following these guidelines will give you a platform from which to experiment:

- Top note oils should make up to 30% of a blend

- Middle note oils should make up to 80% of a blend

- Base note oils should make up to 10% of a blend

Therapeutic blending

This is different from aesthetic blending in that you are trying to achieve a pleasing blend of oils that address specific problems.

Although there are many different oils to choose from it may not be possible always to follow the blending guidelines in order to achieve the right therapeutic blend.

Aromatherapy is an holistic therapy, in other words it addresses the whole person, not just the presenting problem. Every condition will affect an individual physically and psychologically, and the holistic approach will attempt to provide a comprehensive treatment to all aspects of a condition. For example, someone suffering with arthritis may also be feeling depressed. There are several different oils and blends that could be used for arthritis itself, for example Juniperberry and Vetiver, while feelings of depression can be helped with Bergamot, Ylang Ylang, etc. Making a blend using the guidelines above would be perfectly possible with the range of oils available:

> 2 drops Bergamot
> 7 drops Vetiver   } in 20-50 ml of base oil for massage
> 1 drop Ylang Ylang

You will need to test the aroma to check that it is pleasing. You can do this by putting a drop of each oil on a ball of damp cotton wool and trying the fragrance. Adjust as required but do not exceed the total maximum dosage (see Chapter 10, 'General precautions').

In our list of Essential Oils we have indicated those oils that have proved to be very good together in blends. If you find this perplexing and too difficult to follow, a simple rule of blending oils that come from the same family should give you plenty of scope for experimentation:

HERBS - Basil; Chamomile; Clary Sage; Coriander; Fennel; Lavender; Marjoram; Melissa; Peppermint; Rosemary; Spearmint; Thyme

SPICES & CITRUS - Bergamot; Black Pepper; Citronella; Ginger; Grapefruit; Lemon; Lime; Litsea Cubeba; Mandarin; Orange; Tangerine

FLOWERS & GRASSES - Geranium; Jasmine; Lemongrass; Myrtle; Neroli; Palmarosa; Rose; Vetiver; Ylang Ylang

RESINS & TREES - Eucalyptus; Frankincense; Juniperberry;

Myrrh; Niaouli; Patchouli; Petitgrain; Rosewood; Sandalwood; Scots Pine; Tea Tree

Remember - blending is not compulsory! You do not need to use a blend; you will usually find a choice of oils that will help for any particular condition. If you want to experiment and achieve a greater benefit from the result, then go ahead. Be brave and trust your sense of smell and intuition; just make sure that you take note of the general precautions and you will be fine.

Chapter 4

Index of conditions

On the following pages we have listed more than 90 common conditions from which many people suffer, and our recommendations of appropriate oils to use. The first list is a quick-reference index, while the second gives detailed treatment suggestions.

Please remember that for most of the conditions listed there are several other oils that can be used; our list is by no means exhaustive.

Please try our suggestions, but by all means experiment by using our list of Essential Oils (Chapter 6) and following the guidelines there. When you try your own recipes remember to stick to the correct dosage (see Chapter 10, 'General precautions') and choose an appropriate method; using a room burner for a sprain, for example, will not be particularly effective.

When using the same Essential Oil on a day-to-day basis, it is recommend that you alternate between oils for maximum effect, ie if treating the symptoms of insomnia use Lavender for 3 weeks, change to Petitgrain and after a further 3 weeks return to Lavender.

In the treatment suggestions you will see some abbreviations: a 4/10 or 5/10 ratio simply means that you should use 4 or 5 drops of Essential Oil(s) to every 10 millilitres of carrier. Where a massage carrier is mentioned without specifying a certain type you may use whichever you prefer (see 'Carrier oils' in Chapter 2). An 'equal blend' means that the number of drops of two or more Essential Oils should be equal in the blend.

We refer to Evening Primrose blend in the treatment suggestions; you will see from the section on 'Carrier oils' that Evening Primrose should only be used in a 10% blend with another carrier oil.

Quick reference therapeutic index

Usage codes
A Aromatics (room burner); **B** Bath; **C** Conditioner; **F** Footbath;
G Shower gel/liquid soap; **I** Steam inhalation; **L** Lotion; **M** Massage
(full-body or local application); **N** Neat; **P** Compress; **S** Shampoo

Condition	Essential Oils	Usage
Acne	Bergamot, Chamomile, Lavender	B/L/M
Anaemia	Chamomile, Lemon, Sandalwood	B/M
Anxiety	Bergamot, Cedarwood, Coriander, Neroli	A/B/M
Appetite (excess)	Fennel, Patchouli, Rosemary	A/B/M
Appetite (lack of)	Ginger, Lime, Myrrh, Orange, Palmarosa	A/B/M
Arthritis	Ginger, Juniperberry, Lavender, Vetiver	B/L/M/P
Asthma	Cedarwood, Eucalyptus, Lavender, Spearmint	A/B/M
Athlete's foot	Lavender, Patchouli, Tea Tree	B/F/L
Blisters	Lavender	B/L/N
Blood pressure (high)	Lavender, Marjoram, Ylang Ylang	B/L/M
Blood pressure (low)	Clary Sage, Lemon, Rosemary	B/L/M
Body odour	Clary Sage, Lemongrass, Litsea Cubeba, Melissa, Peppermint, Scots Pine	A/B/F/G/L/M
Boils	Chamomile, Lavender, Tea Tree	B/L/M/N/P
Bronchitis	Basil, Cedarwood, Eucalyptus, Myrrh, Myrtle, Sandalwood	A/B/I/M

Usage codes
A Aromatics (room burner); **B** Bath; **C** Conditioner; **F** Footbath;
G Shower gel/liquid soap; **I** Steam inhalation; **L** Lotion; **M** Massage
(full-body or local application); **N** Neat; **P** Compress; **S** Shampoo

Condition	Essential Oils	Usage
Bruises	Black Pepper, Fennel, Lavender, Rosemary	B/L/M/P
Burns (minor)	Chamomile, Eucalyptus, Lavender	B/M
Capillaries (broken)	Chamomile, Lemon	B/L/M
Catarrh	Eucalyptus, Frankincense, Myrrh, Myrtle, Sandalwood	A/B/M
Cellulite	Fennel, Grapefruit, Juniperberry, Thyme	B/M
Chickenpox	Chamomile, Lavender, Tea Tree	B/L/M
Chilblains	Black Pepper, Lemon, Rosemary	B/F/M
Childbirth pains	Jasmine, Lavender	M/P
Cold sores	Bergamot, Eucalyptus, Tea Tree	L/M
Colds	Citronella, Eucalyptus, Niaouli	A/B/I/M
Colic	Chamomile, Lavender, Myrtle	M/P
Constipation	Orange, Rosemary, Spearmint	B/M
Convalescence	Lavender, Lime, Melissa, Rosemary	A/B/M
Corns/calluses	Lemon, Peppermint, Tea Tree	F/M/P
Coughs	Eucalyptus, Myrtle, Sandalwood	A/I/M
Cramp	Citronella, Coriander, Marjoram, Rosemary	B/M/P
Cuts/grazes	Eucalyptus, Lavender, Tea Tree	B/L

Usage codes
A Aromatics (room burner); **B** Bath; **C** Conditioner; **F** Footbath;
G Shower gel/liquid soap; **I** Steam inhalation; **L** Lotion; **M** Massage
(full-body or local application); **N** Neat; **P** Compress; **S** Shampoo

Condition	Essential Oils	Usage
Cystitis	Juniperberry, Lavender, Sandalwood, Tea Tree	B/M/P
Dandruff	Cedarwood, Rosemary, Thyme	C/M/S
Depression	Bergamot, Clary Sage, Lime, Melissa	A/B/M
Dermatitis/ eczema	Chamomile, Geranium, Lavender	B/L/M
Diarrhoea	Chamomile, Coriander, Eucalyptus, Myrrh	M/P
Earache	Chamomile, Lavender	M/P
Fatigue (physical)	Basil, Clary Sage, Geranium, Rosemary	B/M
Fatigue (mental)	Citronella, Grapefruit, Peppermint, Rosemary, Thyme	A/B/M
Flatulence	Basil, Fennel, Litsea Cubeba, Mandarin, Peppermint, Spearmint	B/M
Foot aches	Juniperberry, Lavender, Melissa, Peppermint	F/M
Foot odour	Citronella, Lemongrass, Tea Tree	B/F/M
Frigidity	Basil, Jasmine, Rose, Ylang Ylang	A/B/M
German measles	Chamomile, Eucalyptus, Tea Tree	A
Haemorrhoids	Frankincense, Juniperberry	B/L/M
Hair care	See table in Chapter 5	
Hair loss	Lavender, Palmarosa, Rosemary, Thyme	C/M/S

Usage codes
A Aromatics (room burner); **B** Bath; **C** Conditioner; **F** Footbath;
G Shower gel/liquid soap; **I** Steam inhalation; **L** Lotion; **M** Massage
(full-body or local application); **N** Neat; **P** Compress; **S** Shampoo

Condition	Essential Oils	Usage
Hangover	Fennel, Juniperberry, Myrtle, Orange	A/B/M
Hay fever	Chamomile, Eucalyptus, Juniperberry	A/B/M
Headache	Lavender, Peppermint, Rosemary, Rosewood	A/M/P
Hernia	Ginger, Lavender, Rosemary	B/M
Hyperactivity	Chamomile, Lavender, Ylang Ylang	A/B/M
Impotence	Basil, Coriander, Patchouli, Sandalwood, Ylang Ylang	A/M
Indigestion/ dyspepsia	Coriander, Fennel, Juniperberry, Litsea Cubeba, Peppermint, Tangerine	A/B/M
Influenza	Eucalyptus, Myrrh, Myrtle, Scots Pine, Thyme	A/B/I/M
Insect bites and stings	Citronella, Lavender, Lemon, Tea Tree	L/N/P
Insomnia	Lavender, Neroli, Petitgrain, Tangerine	A/B/M
Lice	Eucalyptus, Geranium, Tea Tree	C/M/S
Lumbago	Basil, Marjoram, Rosemary	B/M/P
Mastitis	Geranium, Lavender, Rosemary	B/M/P
Measles	Chamomile, Eucalyptus, Tea Tree	A
Memory (poor)	Lemon, Palmarosa, Rosemary	A
Menopause	Chamomile, Clary Sage, Geranium	B/M
Migraine	Lavender, Marjoram, Peppermint	A/M/P

Usage codes
A Aromatics (room burner); **B** Bath; **C** Conditioner; **F** Footbath;
G Shower gel/liquid soap; **I** Steam inhalation; **L** Lotion; **M** Massage
(full-body or local application); **N** Neat; **P** Compress; **S** Shampoo

Condition	Essential Oils	Usage
Muscular aches	Basil, Black Pepper, Marjoram, Myrrh, Rosemary, Vetiver	B/M
Nappy rash	Chamomile, Lavender	L/M
Nausea	Fennel, Lavender, Peppermint	A/M
Neuralgia	Chamomile, Citronella, Coriander, Eucalyptus, Marjoram, Thyme	B/P
Nose-bleed	Chamomile, Frankincense, Lemon	P
Periods (heavy)	Geranium, Myrtle, Rose	B/M/P
Periods (irregular)	Chamomile, Clary Sage, Rose, Thyme	B/M/P
Periods (painful)	Basil, Chamomile, Clary Sage, Marjoram	B/M/P
PMT	Chamomile, Clary Sage, Geranium, Rose	A/B/M/P
Pruritis	Chamomile, Lavender, Patchouli	B
Psoriasis	Bergamot, Geranium, Lavender	B/L/M
Rheumatism	Basil, Black Pepper, Coriander, Ginger, Juniperberry, Marjoram	B/M/P
Ringworm	Lavender, Rosemary, Tea Tree	L/S
Sciatica	Chamomile, Juniperberry, Lavender	B/M/P
Shingles	Bergamot, Eucalyptus, Tea Tree	B/M
Sinusitis	Eucalyptus, Niaouli, Scots Pine	A/B
Skin care	See table in Chapter 5	

Usage codes
A Aromatics (room burner); **B** Bath; **C** Conditioner; **F** Footbath;
G Shower gel/liquid soap; **I** Steam inhalation; **L** Lotion; **M** Massage
(full-body or local application); **N** Neat; **P** Compress; **S** Shampoo

Condition	Essential Oils	Usage
Sore throat	Eucalyptus, Lavender, Sandalwood	M/I
Sprains	Black Pepper, Lavender, Marjoram, Rosemary, Vetiver	B/L/P
Stress	Bergamot, Coriander, Myrtle, Neroli, Petitgrain, Spearmint, Ylang Ylang	A/B/M
Sunburn	Chamomile, Lavender, Peppermint	B/L
Tachycardia (palpitations)	Frankincense, Lavender, Neroli, Ylang Ylang	A/B/M
Thrush	Lavender, Lemon, Melissa, Myrrh, Tea Tree	B/M
Tonsillitis	Bergamot, Eucalyptus, Lavender, Sandalwood	A/B/I/M
Travel sickness	Fennel, Lemongrass, Peppermint	B
Varicose veins	Chamomile, Lavender, Lemon	see page 74
Warts and verrucae	Lemon, Tea Tree	F/M/N

Index of conditions and recommended treatments

Condition	Recommended oils	Treatment suggestions
ACNE Over-activity of the sebaceous glands	BERGAMOT CHAMOMILE LAVENDER	Use Chamomile or Lavender neat: 1 or 2 drops on cotton wool. Cleanse area with cotton wool. Treat affected area morning and night until clear. Add 2 drops Bergamot and 3 drops Lavender to 25 ml fragrance-free cleanser and use on affected area daily to keep clear and promote healthy, scar-free skin. Massage body with Rosemary or Geranium to stimulate lymphatic system. *Use half quantity of Essential Oil for facial use.*
ANAEMIA Inadequate oxygen-carrying haemoglobin in the blood	CHAMOMILE LEMON SANDALWOOD	Add 1 drop Sandalwood, 7 drops Chamomile and 2 drops Lemon to 30 ml Sweet Almond base oil and use regularly in a full body massage. Alternatively use 4 drops Lemon in a bath with a fragrance-free bath carrier. Test Lemon on sensitive skins.
ANXIETY A worried or troubled state of mind	BERGAMOT CEDARWOOD CORIANDER NEROLI	Room burner, bath and massage can all be used successfully for Anxiety. Add 2 or 3 drops of any of the recommended oils to a room burner and use regularly; 5 or 6 drops added to a bath will give immediate relief. See STRESS below for further suggestions.

Condition	Recommended oils	Treatment suggestions
APPETITE (EXCESS) Over-eating causing excessive weight gain	FENNEL PATCHOULI ROSEMARY	Massage is the most effective method of treatment for over-eating. Use 2 drops Fennel, 1 drop Patchouli and 1 drop Rosemary in 10 ml base oil. If appetite disturbance is caused by emotional or mental distress treat as ANXIETY or STRESS.
APPETITE (LACK OF) Disturbed eating pattern causing decreased appetite	BERGAMOT CORIANDER GINGER LIME MYRRH ORANGE PALMAROSA	Bath or massage with 2 drops Bergamot, 2 drops Palmarosa and 1 drop Coriander, Lime, Myrrh or Orange all excellent digestive oils and used in Anorexia Nervosa treatments. Use 2/3 drops Lime in a room burner to stimulate the digestive system. Treat daily until appetite is restored.
ARTHRITIS Pain, inflammation and stiffness of the joints	GINGER JUNIPERBERRY LAVENDER VETIVER	Ginger 'warms' the joint, Juniperberry balances the body's chemistry and Lavender reduces pain and inflammation. Use a direct application method, ie massage, bath, cream lotion or compress: 4/5 drops Juniperberry in a bath, or massage with 1 drop Ginger and 4 drops Lavender in 10 ml Jojoba/Sweet Almond base oil. Treat regularly while condition is controlled. When painful or inflamed, use bath, cream or hot compress in the same proportions. Keep joints mobile, but don't force. (See RHEUMATISM)

Condition	Recommended oils	Treatment suggestions
ASTHMA Muscle spasm in the bronchi (lungs) causing breathlessness	CEDARWOOD EUCALYPTUS LAVENDER MYRTLE SPEARMINT	Diet, stress and allergens are all known to cause asthma. The type of asthma is important in terms of treatment. For STRESS see below. Triggers in diet need to be controlled and potential allergens reduced. Regular massage between attacks with 2 drops Cedarwood, 2 drops Lavender and 1 drop Eucalyptus will help. Sniff 2 drops Cedarwood, Myrtle, Spearmint or Eucalyptus on tissue/handkerchief during attack. Steam inhalation may cause congestion, so avoid.
ATHLETE'S FOOT Fungal infection of the foot causing red, flaky skin that is itchy	LAVENDER PATCHOULI TEA TREE	Use bath or foot bath method - 1 drop Patchouli, 3 drops Lavender and 1 drop Tea Tree is a helpful blend. Use 1 or 2 drops Lavender or Tea Tree on cotton wool to wipe affected areas if required. Treat twice daily until clear.
BLISTERS Skin eruption caused by friction or allergic reaction	LAVENDER	DO NOT BURST A BLISTER. Use 2 or 3 drops neat Lavender on cotton wool and wipe carefully over blister. Cover with clean gauze, and prevent further rubbing. Apply neat Lavender to a burst blister and leave uncovered provided there is no risk of infection or further rubbing.

Condition	Recommended oils	Treatment suggestions
BLOOD PRESSURE (HIGH) Hypertension - over-worked heart pumping too much blood through the body	LAVENDER MARJORAM YLANG YLANG	Diet and lifestyle changes as well as Aromatherapy treatment are required. Calming oils and vasodilators are best used for this condition. Using light strokes, massage back and chest with 1 drop Ylang Ylang, 1 drop Lavender and 3 drops Marjoram in 10 ml base of Evening Primrose blend. Treat daily until condition improves, then reduce treatments to twice weekly. Bath, lotion or cream methods can be used.
BLOOD PRESSURE (LOW) Hypotension - insufficient blood being pumped through the body	CLARY SAGE LEMON ROSEMARY THYME	Circulation and heart need to be stimulated to increase blood pressure. Rosemary is one of the most powerful of the stimulant oils for the body's circulation system. Massage back and chest with Rosemary, or use a blend of 1 drop Lemon, 2 drops Clary Sage and 2 drops Rosemary. Add 3 drops Rosemary or Thyme and 1 drop Lemon to a bath, or use lotion or cream. Treat daily until condition improves, then twice weekly.
BODY ODOUR Body chemistry imbalance causing unpleasant aroma	CLARY SAGE LEMONGRASS LITSEA CUBEBA MELISSA PEPPERMINT SCOTS PINE	Bring body back into balance by using 4 drops Juniperberry or Geranium in a bath. Use any of the recommended oils in lotion or cream in a 2/3 drops to 10 ml ratio. Use 4 drops in baths. Blend any permutation up to a maximum of 5 drops to 10 ml base.

Condition	Recommended oils	Treatment suggestions
BOILS Infected and inflamed skin causing pus-filled growths	CHAMOMILE LAVENDER TEA TREE	Since boils take a few days to develop, during which they cause pain and tenderness, use a hot compress of 2 drops Lavender or Chamomile to 'draw out' the boil. Cleanse the area around the boil 2 or 3 times a day with neat Tea Tree on cotton wool. Once burst, use Lavender to help cleanse and heal wound. Keep area clear with daily Tea Tree treatment and use 4 drops Juniperberry in regular baths to de-toxify the system.
BRONCHITIS Inflammation of the main air passages of the lungs (bronchi)	BASIL CEDARWOOD EUCALYPTUS MYRRH MYRTLE SANDALWOOD	Steam inhalation is the best method of treating an acute bronchitis infection. Use 2 or 3 drops Eucalyptus or Sandalwood (or combination) twice daily. Use room burner with any of the recommended oils. Keep warm and rest. Chronic bronchitis may be treated additionally with Basil, Cedarwood, Myrrh or Myrtle in baths, back and chest massage or as above.
BRUISES Blood seeping into tissues from an internal wound	FENNEL LAVENDER ROSEMARY	Use an ice-cold compress with Fennel or Lavender directly on bruised area. Use local massage with Rosemary and Lavender when bruise begins to yellow to stimulate circulation and relieve pain.

Condition	Recommended oils	Treatment suggestions
BURNS (MINOR) Heat causing local destruction of skin layers	CHAMOMILE EUCALYPTUS LAVENDER	Without doubt the most beneficial oil for all types of minor burns is Lavender when applied neat. Use sterile gauze liberally covered with Lavender on larger burns; replace regularly. Chamomile has similar qualities and Eucalyptus is a good analgesic/fever-reducing oil. Remember to use cold running water on all burns before using oils. Do not use lotions or creams on a burn.
CAPILLARIES (BROKEN) Damaged, worn or stretched small blood vessels	CHAMOMILE LEMON MYRTLE	Daily massage of the area with 2 drops Chamomile, 2 drops Myrtle and 1 drop Lemon in 15 ml Peach Kernel base. The same blend in a lotion may also be used. Persevere with this treatment as it will take several weeks before improvement can be seen!
CATARRH Blocked, damaged or infected nasal passages	EUCALYPTUS FRANKINCENSE MYRRH MYRTLE SANDALWOOD	Steam inhalation with 2 or 3 drops of any of the recommended oils. Use 3 drops Eucalyptus, Myrtle or Sandalwood in 10 ml base oil to massage sinuses (either side of nose and above eyes).

Condition	Recommended oils	Treatment suggestions
CELLULITE Fluid retention - build-up of fluid and toxic waste in subcutaneous fat	FENNEL GRAPEFRUIT JUNIPER BERRY	All the recommended oils are excellent for de-toxifying the system. Massage helps to break down the cellulite and allow the oils to work more effectively. A 5 drop/10 ml ratio is advised using a light carrier oil (eg Grapeseed) with either one oil or a blend. Bath with 4 or 5 drops Juniperberry and 1 or 2 drops Fennel or Grapefruit (maximum 6).
CHICKENPOX Varicella - caused by the herpes zoster virus with symptoms of a rash with small red spots that are very itchy and painful	CHAMOMILE LAVENDER TEA TREE	For small children (up to about 4 years old) use 1 or 2 drops Lavender or Chamomile in a bath several times a day to reduce itching and pain. 1 or 2 drops in 10 ml lotion can also be used. For older children the addition of 1 drop Tea Tree will help as it is a major anti-viral oil.
CHILBLAINS Abnormal constriction of surface blood vessels caused by low temperatures	BLACK PEPPER LEMON ROSEMARY	Black Pepper and Rosemary are both vascular oils that will help to improve circulation in the long term. Use 2 drops Black Pepper and 3 drops Lemon in baths or massage. For immediate relief of chilblains use 2 drops Lemon and 3 drops Rosemary in 10 ml carrier to give a vigorous local massage.

Condition	Recommended oils	Treatment suggestions
CHILDBIRTH PAINS Pain during labour affecting many areas	JASMINE LAVENDER	Gentle massage with Lavender or Jasmine over the tummy and lower back will be helpful throughout labour in reducing the pain of contractions. Jasmine is well known as a uterine strengthener and can be used throughout birth and afterwards to aid recovery. A warm compress of Jasmine over the abdomen will be very soothing.
COLD SORES Herpes simplex - a viral infection causing small blisters, usually on the mouth	BERGAMOT EUCALYPTUS TEA TREE	There are many oils that can be used for cold sores. Tea Tree used neat directly on the developing blister will prevent pain and full blister eruption. Use cotton wool to dab area regularly. The other oils can be used in preference or alternately. (See BLISTERS)
COLDS Viral infection causing many varied symptoms	CITRONELLA EUCALYPTUS NIAOULI	Steam inhalation is a very effective treatment - 2 or 3 drops Niaouli or Eucalyptus can be regularly used. Bathing with 2 or 3 drops Citronella will reduce muscular aches and shivers. (See CATARRH and INFLUENZA)

Condition	Recommended oils	Treatment suggestions
COLIC Air or gas trapped in the intestines causing abdominal pain	CHAMOMILE LAVENDER	Usually an infant/childhood problem. 1 or 2 drops of either oil in 10 ml of Peach Kernel can be gently massaged over the child's abdomen. A warm compress of 1 drop of either oil can be used on the abdomen, but remember to keep the child warm and replace the compress regularly until the child calms down again and the pain goes.
CONSTIPATION Compacted waste products causing infrequent or irregular bowel movements	ORANGE ROSEMARY SPEARMINT	Massage of the abdomen is always the best solution for constipation - remember to use clockwise circular strokes. A blend of 1 drop Spearmint, 3 drops Rosemary and 1 drop Orange should be pleasing and effective. Many other oils can be helpful so do experiment as the aroma will be important in that it should not increase nausea. Drink plenty of pure water. A relaxing bath with Bergamot, Lavender or Marjoram can also help.
CONVALESCENCE Transition period from ill health to full recovery	LAVENDER LIME MELISSA ROSEMARY	Lime is one of the most beneficial oils to aid recovery. Use in a bath, room burner or massage. A Rosemary and Lime blend in the convalescent's room burner should encourage appetite and raise spirits, or use a mild blend of Melissa and Lavender massaged into the back and shoulders. (See APPETITE)

Condition	Recommended oils	Treatment suggestions
CORNS/CALLUSES Thickened areas of skin caused by pressure	LEMON PEPPERMINT TEA TREE	Tea Tree and Lemon are both known for their ability to help cure corns and calluses. Use either oil in a foot bath in a relatively strong proportion (3 or 4 drops). Treat twice daily, varying the oils used, until the corn disappears. Peppermint may be added to aid general foot care. Massage and compress methods can also be used. If the callus is on another part of the body (eg the hand), use the other methods and also bath or soak the part of the body affected.
COUGHS Bacterial infection of the throat	EUCALYPTUS MYRTLE SANDALWOOD	Steam inhalation with any of the recommended oils will relieve an exhausting cough (see CATARRH). A throat massage of 2 drops Sandalwood and 3 drops Myrtle in 10 ml of carrier oil is an alternative method. Treat twice daily until the condition clears. Use the recommended oils in a room burner to help, particularly at night.
CRAMP Muscle spasm	CITRONELLA CORIANDER MARJORAM ROSEMARY	Massage with recommended oils singly or in a blend - 5 drops to 10 ml carrier. Keep the area moving. A warm compress can also be applied.

Condition	Recommended oils	Treatment suggestions
CUTS/GRAZES Surface wounds causing bleeding	EUCALYPTUS LAVENDER TEA TREE	Clean the area with warm water. Add 2 or 3 drops Lavender or Tea Tree to more water and carefully bathe the area. Cover the wound with gauze that has had 2 or 3 drops Lavender added. Replace dressing at least twice a day. Eucalyptus can also be used if preferred as it is a major analgesic and anti-bacterial.
CYSTITIS Infection of the bladder causing inflammation and pain on passing urine	JUNIPERBERRY LAVENDER SANDALWOOD TEA TREE	Avoid sugar, strong foods and alcohol. Drink plenty of water. Use Juniperberry regularly in a bath while affected to expel toxins. Lavender in a sitz bath or as a genital wash can be used after painful passing of urine to relieve pain and soreness. A blend of 3 drops Juniperberry and 2 drops Sandalwood in a bath is a useful urinary antiseptic. Massage with Sandalwood and Lavender over the lower abdomen will reduce pain, and a hot compress over the same area could also be used. If in doubt of diagnosis always seek medical advice.
DANDRUFF Abnormal production of dead skin cells on the scalp	CEDARWOOD ROSEMARY THYME	Massage the scalp with 2 drops Cedarwood in 5 ml Jojoba carrier oil daily. Use Rosemary or Thyme in massage to stimulate circulation or put 2 drops in the final rinse when washing hair. Use gentle shampoo.

Condition	Recommended oils	Treatment suggestions
DEPRESSION Transient feeling of hopelessness and misery	BERGAMOT CLARY SAGE LIME MELISSA	The type of depression and symptoms experienced will determine which oils to use. If restless and irritable, use Clary Sage, Sandalwood or Ylang Ylang. If withdrawn and lethargic, use Bergamot, Lime, Mandarin, etc. Massage is an excellent method, but all the others can be beneficial. Find which blend of oils appeals most.
DERMATITIS/ECZEMA Itchy inflammation of the skin of many types and several causes	CHAMOMILE GERANIUM LAVENDER	This condition responds well to lotions or creams as well as baths and massage. Use 2 drops Lavender or Chamomile with 2 drops Geranium in 10 ml Wheatgerm and Grapeseed or Evening Primrose and Sweet Almond for massage or in 10 ml lotion/cream. Blend any of these oils, or many others, for baths. Use twice a day during attacks and regularly at other times. *Use half quantity of Essential Oil for facial use.*
DIARRHOEA Passing abnormal and excessive amounts of mostly liquid faecal matter	CHAMOMILE CORIANDER EUCALYPTUS MYRRH	If the result of a virus, diarrhoea will respond well to Eucalyptus. When caused by emotional trauma use Chamomile. Coriander is an excellent anti-spasmodic that will reduce stomach spasms. Massage with 5 drops oil to 10 ml carrier. A warm compress can be used on the abdomen to reduce pain. Drink water.

Condition	Recommended oils	Treatment suggestions
EARACHE Infection of the outer, middle or inner ear - usually a secondary infection	CHAMOMILE LAVENDER	Treat with care, and use only Chamomile or Lavender to treat the ears. Massage around the ear with 1 drop Lavender and 1 drop Chamomile in 5 ml Sweet Almond. Use a warm compress of the same oils to draw out any infection. Place a couple of drops of the blend on some cotton wool and place carefully in the ear; remove after 1 or 2 hours. If symptoms persist we suggest that a medical diagnosis is sought.
FATIGUE (PHYSICAL) Extreme physical tiredness - exhaustion	BASIL CLARY SAGE GERANIUM ROSEMARY	Massage and bath are the best two methods to regenerate and energise. Use 3 or 4 drops Clary Sage in a bath, or massage with equal amounts of Geranium and Rosemary in carrier oil (4 drops to 10 ml). Basil, Marjoram and Orange are other oils very useful for physical fatigue.
FATIGUE (MENTAL) Extreme lassitude or listlessness - inability to concentrate	CITRONELLA GRAPEFRUIT PEPPERMINT ROSEMARY	Together with massage and bath, the room burner method is effective in revitalising the mind. Use Grapefruit on its own in a bath (4 drops) or room burner. A blend of 3 drops Rosemary and 1 drop Peppermint in a carrier oil for massage is recommended. There are many other stimulant oils that you may wish to try.

Condition	Recommended oils	Treatment suggestions
FLATULENCE Expelling of gas from the digestive system caused by inhaled air, food or anxiety	BASIL FENNEL LITSEA CUBEBA MANDARIN PEPPERMINT SPEARMINT	Any of the carminative oils can be used for this condition. Massage over the abdomen with any one of these oils or a blend of 2 or 3 different oils. Use a 4 drop/10 ml dilution and use light circular movements around the abdomen. 4 or 5 drops of oil in a bath will also help. (See INDIGESTION)
FOOT ACHES General aches or inflammation of the foot	JUNIPERBERRY LAVENDER MELISSA PEPPERMINT	Peppermint is renowned for its ability to refresh and revitalise tired, aching feet - use 2 or 3 drops in a footbath. Massage of the feet is beneficial for the whole and particularly good for aching feet. The three oils recommended in a blend of 5 drops to 10 ml carrier will bring immediate relief. (See MUSCULAR ACHES)
FOOT ODOUR Excessive sweating or a fungal infection	CITRONELLA LEMONGRASS TEA TREE	If caused by a fungal infection use Tea Tree in a footbath or bath - 3 drops should be sufficient - but if you dislike the aroma of Tea Tree add 1 drop of Patchouli or a drop of a citrus oil. Lemongrass, along with several other oils, are excellent deodorants that can be used in both baths or massage for excessive sweating.

Condition	Recommended oils	Treatment suggestions
FRIGIDITY Inability of women to achieve orgasm	BASIL JASMINE ROSE YLANG YLANG	Sexual response depends on many things - frigidity is not the inability to function sexually, but the inability to enjoy it! Mood, approach, circumstances and environment will all make a difference (see STRESS/ANXIETY). Apart from those listed there are several other aphrodisiac oils, eg Patchouli and Rosewood. Massage, bath and room burner are all good methods of using these oils singly or in a blend of 2 or 3 different oils.
GERMAN MEASLES Rubella - a contagious viral infection with cold-like symptoms - not as severe as Measles	CHAMOMILE EUCALYPTUS TEA TREE	Keep the sick room free of the virus by using a room burner with 2 or 3 drops Eucalyptus or Tea Tree (depending on patient's age!). A room spray can also be used. Sponge the patient once daily with 4 drops Chamomile in 1 pint of tepid water to reduce fever. Other symptoms may be treated separately.
HAEMORRHOIDS Anal varicose veins - swollen, twisted and thin-walled veins	FRANKINCENSE JUNIPERBERRY MYRTLE	A blend of 2 drops Frankincense, 2 drops Myrtle and 1 drop Juniperberry can be added to a bath and taken regularly when haemorrhoids are painful. Apply the same blend in a lotion directly to haemorrhoids regularly. Use Lavender on cotton pads after going to the toilet.

Condition	Recommended oils	Treatment suggestions
HAIR LOSS Thinning or loss of hair on all or part of the head	LAVENDER PALMAROSA ROSEMARY THYME	Rosemary has for centuries been the choice for hair loss. Use 2 drops in the final rinse after washing hair. Alternatively make an alcohol rub for the scalp: add 2 drops Rosemary or Thyme to 5 ml alcohol (high-proof vodka is best) and massage into scalp regularly. Alopecia can be treated with 2 drops Lavender and 2 drops Palmarosa in 10 ml Evening Primrose and Sweet Almond or Jojoba and Sweet Almond. Massage into the scalp, leave for 30 minutes then shampoo.
HANGOVER Build-up of toxic waste causing various symptoms	FENNEL JUNIPERBERRY ORANGE	Bath, room burner and massage are good methods for hangovers. Use 1 drop Orange and 4 drops Juniperberry in a bath. Massage with 1 drop Orange and 4 drops Fennel in 10 ml carrier. Add 3 or 4 drops of Fennel or Juniperberry to a room burner.
HAY FEVER Allergic rhinitis - inflammation and fluid retention in the eyes, nose and throat caused by airborne irritants	CHAMOMILE EUCALYPTUS JUNIPERBERRY	Put 1 or 2 drops Eucalyptus on a tissue/hankie and sniff regularly to keep clear. Use Juniperberry in a bath or massage. 1 drop Eucalyptus and 3 drops Chamomile in a room burner will create a beneficial atmosphere. Use the same blend in 10 ml carrier to massage sinuses. (See COLDS)

Condition	Recommended oils	Treatment suggestions
HEADACHE (TENSION) Strain on the muscular tissues or blood vessels in the head or neck	LAVENDER PEPPERMINT ROSEMARY ROSEWOOD	Massage with Lavender alone or 2 drops Lavender and 2 drops Peppermint in 10 ml carrier around the back of the neck, temples and forehead. Use Rosemary to help blood flow and clear the head in 4/10 ratio. Rub 2 drops Lavender neat into the temples or put on to a cold compress and place on the temples, forehead or back of the neck. The use of any of the oils in a room burner may also be beneficial. (See STRESS, COLDS, MIGRAINE)
HEADACHE (NAUSEA) As above but accompanied by actual vomiting or feelings of nausea	LAVENDER PEPPERMINT ROSEWOOD	Treat as above but massage of the abdomen with Rosewood alone or in an equal 4/10 blend with Peppermint should also give relief. Use the same blend in a bath. With headaches don't be tempted to overdose as this will make the condition worse not better! (See NAUSEA)
HERNIA Bulge of soft tissue that protrudes through a muscle wall - usually abdominal	GINGER LAVENDER ROSEMARY	Massage over the abdomen and lower back with 2 drops Ginger, 2 drops Lavender and 1 drop Rosemary in 10 ml carrier oil daily when painful and swollen. Regular use of this blend afterwards will help. The same blend can be used in a bath.

Condition	Recommended oils	Treatment suggestions
HYPERACTIVITY Physical and mental restlessness in children with poor attention, tantrums and little need of sleep	CHAMOMILE LAVENDER YLANG YLANG	Use only Chamomile or Lavender on children under 4 years old; Ylang Ylang may be added for older children. Massage, bath and room burner are the most effective methods. Use 2 drops of either oil in 10 ml Evening Primrose blend for daily back massage; 2 or 3 drops in the bath will also be calming. Use 2 drops in a room burner in the child's room at night to aid sleep.
IMPOTENCE Inability of men to achieve or maintain an erection	BASIL CORIANDER PATCHOULI SANDALWOOD YLANG YLANG	Massage the whole body with 5 drops of one or a blend of the oils in 10 ml carrier. Use aphrodisiac and sedative oils to relax and instil confidence. Other oils include Coriander, Jasmine, Neroli and Rosewood. A bath with the same oils will also be effective, and use of the room burner will help.
INDIGESTION/ DYSPEPSIA General sense of discomfort in the abdomen - sharp, dull or gnawing pain in the chest	CORIANDER FENNEL JUNIPERBERRY LITSEA CUBEBA PEPPERMINT TANGERINE	Use the recommended oils in a massage over the abdomen. A blend of 2 drops Fennel or Peppermint and 2 drops Juniperberry in 10 ml carrier will help. Use the same oils in a bath as an alternative. (See CONSTIPATION/ FLATULENCE)

Condition	Recommended oils	Treatment suggestions
INFLUENZA Viral infection causing a variety of respiratory and muscular symptoms	EUCALYPTUS MYRRH MYRTLE SCOTS PINE THYME	Bath, massage, inhalation and room burner can all be used for this condition. Daily baths with 1 drop Myrrh, 3 drops Scots Pine and 2 drops Eucalyptus or 2 drops Thyme and 3 drops Myrtle should be taken. Use Eucalyptus or Scots Pine in an inhalation 3 times a day. Use either oil in a room burner in the patient's room regularly. (See other similar conditions)
INSECT BITES AND STINGS Local itching and swelling causing pain	CITRONELLA LAVENDER LEMON TEA TREE	Apply Lavender or Tea Tree neat to the affected area. 1 or 2 drops on cotton wool dabbed on the area will clean, relieve pain and promote skin healing. A cold compress of 1 drop Lemon and 2 drops Lavender will help to stop bleeding and reduce swelling. Use Citronella, Lemongrass and Peppermint to prevent insect bites and stings.
INSOMNIA Frequent difficulty in falling or staying asleep during the night	LAVENDER NEROLI PETITGRAIN TANGERINE	Most of the sedative oils will be helpful in promoting a good night's sleep. Lavender in a room burner, bath or massage before retiring is very effective; alternate with Neroli or Petitgrain. Blend oils to a maximum of 4/10 ratio to find a pleasing aroma for the individual.

Condition	Recommended oils	Treatment suggestions
LICE Tiny insects living in the hair and sucking blood from the skin, causing irritation	EUCALYPTUS GERANIUM TEA TREE	Blend 1 drop Eucalyptus, 1 drop Tea Tree and 2 drops Geranium in 10 ml Sweet Almond. Massage into infected area and leave for 2 or 3 hours. Wash with a fragrance-free shampoo/shower gel and comb through the hair with a fine-toothed comb. Repeat the treatment every 2 days until clear. Remember to clean bedding, clothing, collars, scarves, etc, to remove the eggs.
LUMBAGO Pain in the lumbar region of the back caused by unusual exertion	BASIL MARJORAM ROSEMARY	Rest the back. Massage, compress and bath can all be used for this condition. Use a hot compress with 1 drop Basil, 2 drops Rosemary and 2 drops Marjoram added. Place on the lumbar area and keep warm. Massage with the same blend in 10 ml carrier over the lumbar area or use in a bath. Treat twice daily until the pain is relieved. (See MUSCULAR ACHES)
MASTITIS Breast abscess - a red, tender swelling or lump in the breast	GERANIUM LAVENDER ROSEMARY	Treatment should aim to reduce swelling and relieve pain, as for any abscess. Use a tepid compress of Lavender alone or a blend of 1 drop of each oil. A bath using any one or a blend of these oils will help. Rest in bed and treat regularly.

Condition	Recommended oils	Treatment suggestions
MEASLES Highly contagious viral infection mainly affecting the skin and respiratory tract with flu-like symptoms, diarrhoea, spots and rash; sometimes headaches and sensitivity to light are experienced	CHAMOMILE EUCALYPTUS TEA TREE	Treat as for German Measles, but this condition is much more serious and contagious. Treatment must be continuous and regular throughout the illness. Continuous vaporisation in the patient's room by room burner and spray is recommended - use Tea Tree or Eucalyptus for this purpose. Regular sponging of the whole body with Chamomile to reduce fever is vital. (See GERMAN MEASLES and other similar conditions)
MEMORY (POOR) Difficulty in remembering individual events and facts - absent-mindedness	LEMON PALMAROSA ROSEMARY	These oils are known for their ability to clarify the mind and aid concentration. Use in a room burner individually or as a blend of 3 or 4 drops.
MENOPAUSE Transition period for women during which hormonal changes can cause a variety of disturbances	CHAMOMILE CLARY SAGE GERANIUM	This is not an individual condition as such and therefore each symptom can be addressed separately. For general help during this period a regular massage and bath using one or a blend of the recommended oils will help. Use a 4/10 ratio in Evening Primrose blend carrier for massage and in the bath. (See other similar conditions)

Condition	Recommended oils	Treatment suggestions
MIGRAINE Sever headache caused by restricted blood supply to the head	LAVENDER MARJORAM PEPPERMINT	We advise that you do not attempt to treat a migraine attack once it has fully developed - prevention when the first signs of an attack are detected is better. Treat as headaches using massage of the temples and cold compresses. Blood supply can be encouraged by the use of Marjoram in a warm compress on the back of the neck. (See HEADACHES)
MUSCULAR ACHES General aches and pains of voluntary muscles	BASIL BLACK PEPPER MARJORAM MYRRH ROSEMARY VETIVER	General aches and pains in the muscles can be caused by many things. A general tonic for aching muscles is a massage with 1 drop Basil, 2 drops Rosemary and 2 drops Marjoram in 10 ml carrier. Use a blend in the bath. Treat daily until aches or pains are relieved. Oils can be used individually if preferred and several other anti-spasmodic oils can be used. (See other similar conditions)
NAPPY RASH Skin inflammation caused by various irritants, eg urine, faeces, soap, detergent, etc	CHAMOMILE LAVENDER	Thoroughly wash the area. Use cotton wool dipped in a bowl of warm water with 1 drop of each oil added to wipe over the area. Pat dry thoroughly. Add 1 drop each of the oils to 10 ml fragrance-free lotion or cream and apply to the area. Repeat twice daily until the condition clears.

Condition	Recommended oils	Treatment suggestions
NAUSEA General feeling of sickness or actual vomiting - many causes	FENNEL LAVENDER PEPPERMINT	Nausea is usually associated with other conditions, eg headaches. For general unspecific feelings of nausea use recommended oils individually or blended in a massage (4/10) over the abdomen. Make sure that the aroma of the blend is pleasing or this may itself cause nausea! (See other similar conditions)
NEURALGIA Sharp pain from a damaged nerve	CHAMOMILE CITRONELLA CORIANDER EUCALYPTUS MARJORAM THYME	Powerful analgesic and nervine oils are needed. Use the recommended oils, individually or blended, twice daily while in pain. A hot compress over the affected part of the body is the best method of treating neuralgia. Use the oils in a bath as an alternative. Use 2 or 3 drops in a compress and up to 6 drops in a bath.
NOSE-BLEED Sudden bleeding from the nose, usually caused by damaged nasal linings	CHAMOMILE FRANKINCENSE LEMON	Lemon is probably the best haemostatic (stops bleeding) oil. A cold compress of Chamomile and/or Frankincense can be placed on the back of the neck and the patient should sit with the head forward, allowing the blood to flow out of the nose until the bleeding stops. If the bleeding continues for 30 minutes, seek medical advice.

Condition	Recommended oils	Treatment suggestions
PERIODS (HEAVY) Menorrhagia - prolonged periods with excessive bleeding	GERANIUM MYRTLE ROSE	Bath, compress and massage are all suitable methods to use for any period (menstruation) problems. Use 1 drop Rose, 2 drops Geranium and 2 drops Myrtle in 10 ml Evening Primrose blended carrier for twice-daily massage over the abdomen and groin. Use oils separately or in a blend for baths. A hot compress using single or blended oils can be used to ease pain. **Avoid all Emmenagogue oils** (see page 88), although the benefits of Rose appear to outweigh any minor emmenagogue effects in this instance.
PERIODS (IRREGULAR) Amenorrhea - scanty and infrequent periods	CHAMOMILE CLARY SAGE ROSE THYME	Help to increase regularity is needed here - Chamomile and Clary Sage are both good oils to stimulate blood production during menstruation. Use 1 drop Rose, 2 drops Clary Sage and 2 drops Chamomile as a blend, or use the oils individually. Methods as above.
PERIODS (PAINFUL) Dysmenorrhoea - various sites of dull pain before and during periods	BASIL CHAMOMILE CLARY SAGE MARJORAM	In general the most common problem during menstruation is pain. Methods as above covering the lower back as well as the abdomen. Use 1 drop Clary Sage and 2 drops Basil, Chamomile and Marjoram as a blend, or use oils individually.

Condition	Recommended oils	Treatment suggestions
PMT Hormonal changes causing physical, mental and emotional disturbance	CHAMOMILE CLARY SAGE GERANIUM ROSE	Massage, daily during the week before menstruation, with the recommended oils will reduce PMT symptoms. Use 1 drop Rose and 2 drops each Chamomile and Geranium in full body or abdomen and lower back massage. Baths and hot compresses can also help symptoms. Carry a tissue with 1 or 2 drops of Rose to sniff throughout the day to soothe emotions.
PRURITUS Fungal infection in the groin, armpit or anus; head can also be affected - ringworm	CHAMOMILE LAVENDER PATCHOULI	This is a similar condition to Athlete's foot in other parts of the body. Keep the affected area as clean and dry as possible. Wash the area regularly with 2 drops Lavender or Chamomile added to 5 ml vodka and half a pint of cool water. When clear keep it so by applying (not massage) 1 drop Patchouli and 2 drops Lavender or Chamomile in 10 ml Sweet Almond carrier. (See ATHLETE'S FOOT)
PSORIASIS Speeded-up production of new skin cells preventing production of keratin causing unsightly flaky skin; slight itching or soreness may occur	BERGAMOT GERANIUM LAVENDER	Make up a fragrance-free lotion consisting of 1 drop Bergamot, 2 drops Geranium and 1 drop Lavender in 10 ml lotion. Apply liberally to the affected areas. The recommended oils can be used in a bath or lightly massaged into the skin using Evening Primrose blended or Wheatgerm blended carriers. (See DERMATITIS)

Condition	Recommended oils	Treatment suggestions
RHEUMATISM Diseased muscles become inflamed, swollen and painful	BASIL BLACK PEPPER CORIANDER GINGER JUNIPERBERRY MARJORAM	Massage as often as possible over the whole body and particularly the affected muscles. Use recommended oils individually - Juniperberry to eliminate toxins and Basil, Ginger and Marjoram to relieve muscular pains. Use 4 drops in 1 ml Olive oil and 9 ml Grapeseed or Sweet Almond. Hot compresses using Ginger or Marjoram may be used over the affected muscles. (See ARTHRITIS)
RINGWORM Fungal infection causing scaly, itchy patches on scalp or body	LAVENDER ROSEMARY TEA TREE	Use 3 or 4 drops Lavender or Tea Tree in a fragrance-free cream or lotion and apply to the affected areas several times a day. Blend both oils equally if you wish. Use 2 drops Rosemary in hair rinses to promote hair growth when the infection is cleared. (See ATHLETE'S FOOT)
SCIATICA Pain caused by pressure on the sciatic nerve running from the groin down the leg	CHAMOMILE JUNIPERBERRY LAVENDER	Baths and warm compresses can help ease the pain of Sciatica. A light massage with 2 drops Lavender and 1 each Chamomile and Juniperberry in 10 ml carrier can be used over the affected area. Use Chamomile or Lavender in a warm compress regularly. (See NEURALGIA)

Condition	Recommended oils	Treatment suggestions
SHINGLES Herpes zoster - viral infection of the same family as chickenpox; nerves are infected, and painful skin blisters follow affected nerve	BERGAMOT EUCALYPTUS TEA TREE	Baths are probably the easiest way of treating Shingles. Use 3 drops Eucalyptus and 3 drops Bergamot in baths regularly when painful. Blisters can be treated by using a soft paintbrush: make up a blend of 2 drops Tea Tree and 2 drops Bergamot in 10 ml vodka or Sweet Almond and paint the blend over the blisters several times a day. Use Bergamot in a room burner to reduce stress. (See CHICKENPOX)
SINUSITIS Inflammation of the sinuses from bacterial or viral infection	EUCALYPTUS NIAOULI SCOTS PINE	Steam inhalations several times a day should be used to treat Sinusitis. Use 2 or 3 drops of the recommended oils alternately. A room burner with any of the oils will be helpful in maintaining the attack on the virus. Baths can be used, and if there is fever the Eucalyptus should be preferred. (See COLDS, INFLUENZA)
SORE THROAT Rough or raw feeling in the back of the throat causing discomfort	EUCALYPTUS LAVENDER SANDALWOOD	Steam inhalations using 2 or 3 drops Eucalyptus several times daily until the condition clears. Add 1 or 2 drops Lavender to attack any viruses present. Use 2 drops Sandalwood in 5 ml carrier to massage the throat. (See TONSILLITIS)

Condition	Recommended oils	Treatment suggestions
SPRAINS Torn or damaged ligaments causing pain and tenderness	BLACK PEPPER LAVENDER MARJORAM ROSEMARY VETIVER	Do not massage a sprain. Use a cold compress with Black Pepper, Lavender, Marjoram and Vetiver added and keep the joint rested. Add 2 drops Rosemary and Lavender to 10 ml fragrance-free lotion and apply to the area when the swelling and pain have reduced.
STRESS Substantial change to the normal demands on one's mental and emotional resources	BERGAMOT CORIANDER MYRTLE NEROLI PETITGRAIN SPEARMINT YLANG YLANG	There are many sedative and relaxing oils that can be used to help with Stress. Massage is by far the best method to use. Blend oils of your choice in a 5/10 ratio so that a pleasing aroma is achieved. A blend of 1 drop Neroli, 3 drops Petitgrain and 1 drop Bergamot should please most people. (See ANXIETY)
SUNBURN Inflammation of the skin caused by over-exposure to ultraviolet rays	CHAMOMILE LAVENDER PEPPERMINT	Get as much heat out of the skin as possible by bathing or showering in cold water (unless the skin is blistering). Add 4 drops Lavender to half a pint of ice-cold water and dab liberally over the burnt area with cotton pads or wool. When heat and pain are under control a blend of 4 drops Lavender and 1 drop Peppermint can be used in 10 ml of fragrance-free lotion and applied. Alternatively add the blend to a bath.

Condition	Recommended oils	Treatment suggestions
TACHYCARDIA (PALPITATIONS) Over-rapid heartbeat causing shortness of breath and faintness	FRANKINCENSE LAVENDER NEROLI YLANG YLANG	For immediate relief put 2 or 3 drops Ylang Ylang on a tissue and sniff when experiencing palpitations. Regular massage using any of the recommended oils will help to regulate the heartbeat. Use in 4/10 ratio with any suitable carrier, and blend to please. Also use oils in the bath. (See STRESS)
THRUSH Candida albicans - fungal growths in either the mouth or vagina causing soreness, irritation and pain	LAVENDER LEMON MELISSA MYRRH TEA TREE	Baths with 3 drops Tea Tree (alternatively Melissa or Myrrh) and 1 drop Lemon can reduce the fungal infection. Use Lavender if Tea Tree irritates your skin, and Lemon can be left out. 2 or 3 drops Lavender added to half a pint of warm water can be used as a local wash after passing urine. Diet will have a significant impact on Thrush and Stress will not help. (See CYSTITIS)
TONSILLITIS Acute infection of the tonsils causing flu-like symptoms	BERGAMOT EUCALYPTUS LAVENDER SANDALWOOD	Steam inhalation with Eucalyptus (2 drops) and Lavender (2 drops) will fight infection and reduce inflammation. Use several times a day while the condition persists. Use Bergamot in a bath to relax and soothe. (See SORE THROAT, INFLUENZA)

Condition	Recommended oils	Treatment suggestions
TRAVEL SICKNESS Symptoms as Nausea, caused by motion	FENNEL LEMONGRASS PEPPERMINT	Travel sickness can be treated as Nausea. Add 1 or 2 drops of any of the recommended oils to a tissue/hankie, and sniff regularly while travelling. A bath with Bergamot or Neroli before travelling will reduce stress, and palpitations caused by anxiety can be treated as above. (See NAUSEA, STRESS, ANXIETY, TACHYCARDIA)
VARICOSE VEINS Damaged and worn veins or valves in the veins restricting the return of blood to the heart	CHAMOMILE LAVENDER LEMON	Do not massage below or over varicose veins. Gently massage with a 4/10 ratio of Chamomile regularly. Add 3 drops Chamomile or Lavender and 1 drop Lemon to 10 ml cream and apply daily to the affected area. Warm compresses of Chamomile or Lavender will also help. Rest with the legs higher than the head. Gentle stretching exercises will help. Don't expect immediate relief - it may take some time. Treat daily. (See BLOOD PRESSURE)
WARTS AND VERRUCAE Viral infection causing skin cells to multiply and produce small, hard growths; usually painless	LEMON ROSEMARY TEA TREE	Use neat Lemon or Tea Tree alternately; 1 drop placed directly on the wart or verruca, then covered with a dry plaster. Repeat daily until the condition disappears. After it has gone massage the area with 10 ml Wheatgerm blended carrier and 4 drops Rosemary or Lavender.

Chapter 5

Skin and hair care

*E*ssential Oils should not be kept just for when you are ill. One of the most enjoyable ways of using Essential Oils is in daily hair and body care. Using fragrance-free lotions, creams, moisturisers, cleansers, toners, shampoos and conditioners, you can create a range of cosmetics and toiletries for your particular skin and hair and with your favourite aromas. For the whole body use a fragrance-free bath carrier and shower gel to complete your range. You need to make sure that the products you use are lanolin-free (lanolin is derived from sheep's wool and will not penetrate the skin) as this has been known to cause reactions in some people's skin.

Essential Oils are excellent for all types of skin as they all have some property that affects it. There are oils that are good as anti-ageing agents; others that help prevent wrinkles; most will stimulate skin cell renewal; and others are good as bactericides or anti-inflammatories.

Hair can also be treated with Essential Oils. Any specific hair conditions, for example dandruff and hair loss, are listed in Chapter 4. There are several choices of oils you can use to wash and condition regularly different types of hair and keep it in peak condition.

Skin care

Do you know what sort of skin you have? Most of us are not too sure, so here are a few clues:

Dry skin often looks thin and feels tight. It is prone to dry patches and flaking, fine lines and wrinkles. Dry skin is usually sensitive and tends to age more quickly than other skin types.

Normal skin looks clear and feels neither tight nor greasy. Although the odd spot might appear, it is generally blemish-free.

Oily skin looks and feels greasy after cleansing. It is prone to blackheads and spots, and often looks sallow and dull or lifeless.

Sensitive skin is often fair and translucent with scarcely visible pores, and may also be fragile and easily torn. It will usually react strongly to heat and cold, causing it to become dry and taut; it can become painful with redness, blotching and even itching.

Mature skin is characterised by loss of elasticity and will not return to its natural shape very quickly when pinched. Fine lines and wrinkles appear, particularly at the eyes and mouth. Mature skin tends to be fragile and tears easily. It is also thin and translucent.

Combination skin, as the name suggests, will tend to vary across small areas from oily to dry. Some people have patchy skin, while others can have what are called 'panels' of different types of skin across parts of the body. Try to treat individual areas, particularly if you have panels, but otherwise treat as for the majority skin type you have.

Routine
In order to keep your skin healthy and looking good you must establish a regular routine and maintain it:

Nightly Cleanse face and neck
Apply toner with cotton wool
Put night cream or moisturiser on face and neck

Daily Cleanse if required
Wipe face and neck with toner on cotton wool
Apply moisturiser

Weekly Massage the face and neck
(see 'Methods of use' in Chapter 2)

You can use fragrance-free lotion as an alternative to moisturiser.

Don't forget the rest of the body - this needs care as well as the face and neck - use lotion, moisturiser and cream regularly. Massages, baths and showers should also be used regularly to rejuvenate the skin. You can also make your own hand creams using a fragrance-free cream with added Essential Oils. Use the same Essential Oils as detailed below for each particular hand skin type.

Remember - for facial care we recommend a maximum dilution of 1 drop of Essential Oil for every 5 ml or 5 g of base. For adult bodycare the maximum dosage is 5 drops to 10 ml or 10 g of base. Always begin by using the lowest dosage, ie 1 drop for every 5 ml or 5 g base.

Skin care Essential Oils by skin type

Dry
Chamomile; Frankincense; Geranium; Jasmine; Lavender; Myrrh; Neroli; Palmarosa; Patchouli; Rose; Rosemary; Rosewood; Sandalwood; Ylang Ylang
Massage carriers: All, particularly Wheatgerm

Normal
Chamomile; Fennel; Frankincense; Geranium; Lavender; Lemon; Neroli; Patchouli; Rose; Rosewood; Sandalwood; Ylang Ylang
Massage carriers: All

Oily
Bergamot; Cedarwood; Citronella; Fennel; Geranium; Jasmine; Juniperberry; Lavender; Lemon; Lemongrass; Lime; Litsea Cubeba; Myrtle; Orange; Patchouli; Peppermint; Rosewood; Spearmint; Tangerine; Tea Tree; Thyme; Vetiver; Ylang Ylang
Massage carriers: Peach Kernel; Grapeseed, Jojoba

Sensitive
Chamomile; Jasmine; Lavender; Myrrh; Myrtle; Neroli; Palmarosa; Peppermint; Rose; Rosewood; Sandalwood; Tangerine; Ylang Ylang
Massage carriers: Evening Primrose; Peach Kernel

Mature
Basil; Cedarwood; Fennel; Frankincense; Geranium; Lavender;
Myrrh; Neroli; Orange; Palmarosa; Patchouli; Rose; Rosewood;
Sandalwood
Massage carriers: Evening Primrose; Peach Kernel

Combination
Cedarwood; Chamomile; Geranium; Jasmine; Juniperberry;
Lavender; Myrrh; Rosewood; Sandalwood; Tea Tree; Thyme; Ylang
Ylang
Massage carriers: All

Skin care Essential Oils by oil

	Dry	Normal	Oily	Sensitive	Mature	Combi- nation
BASIL					●	
BERGAMOT			●			
CEDARWOOD			●		●	●
CHAMOMILE	●	●		●		●
CITRONELLA			●			
FENNEL		●	●		●	
FRANKINCENSE	●	●			●	
GERANIUM	●	●	●		●	●
JASMINE	●		●	●		●
JUNIPERBERRY			●			●
LAVENDER	●	●	●	●	●	●
LEMON		●	●			
LEMONGRASS			●			
LIME			●			
LITSEA CUBEBA			●			
MYRRH	●			●	●	●
MYRTLE			●	●		

	Dry	Normal	Oily	Sensitive	Mature	Combi-nation
NEROLI	●	●		●	●	
ORANGE			●		●	
PALMAROSA	●			●	●	
PATCHOULI	●	●	●		●	
PEPPERMINT				●	●	
ROSE	●	●		●	●	
ROSEMARY	●					
ROSEWOOD	●	●	●	●	●	●
SANDALWOOD	●	●		●	●	●
SPEARMINT			●			
TANGERINE			●	●		
TEA TREE			●			●
THYME			●			●
VETIVER			●			
YLANG YLANG	●	●	●	●		●

Recipes
The following recipes are all total drops if using 25 ml or g of base. For baths, showers and massage, see 'Methods of use' in Chapter 2.

Dry skin
Cleanser: 2 drops Sandalwood and 3 drops Rosewood
Toner: 3 drops Frankincense and 2 drops Palmarosa
Moisturiser: 2 drops Ylang Ylang and 3 drops Geranium
Bath/shower: 2 drops Frankincense and 4 drops Lavender
Massage: 1 drop Patchouli, 2 drops Neroli and 2 drops Palmarosa

Normal skin
Cleanser: 2 drops Lemon and 3 drops Chamomile
Toner: 2 drops Sandalwood and 3 drops Fennel
Moisturiser: 4 drops Geranium and 1 drop Patchouli

Bath/shower: 2 drops Lemon and 4 drops Ylang Ylang
Massage: 2 drops Rose and 3 drops Geranium

Oily skin
Cleanser: 3 drops Bergamot and 2 drops Lime
Toner: 3 drops Myrtle and 2 drops Peppermint
Moisturiser: 2 drops Orange and 3 drops Juniperberry
Bath/shower: 2 drops Cedarwood, 3 drops Juniperberry and 1 drop Lemon
Massage: 3 drops Juniperberry and 2 drops Lemongrass

Sensitive skin
Cleanser: 2 drops Sandalwood and 3 drops Rosewood
Toner: 2 drops Peppermint and 3 drops Lavender
Moisturiser: 2 drops Ylang Ylang and 3 drops Chamomile
Bath/shower: 3 drops Lavender and 3 drops Chamomile
Massage: 3 drops Neroli and 2 drops Lavender

Mature/ageing skin
Cleanser: 3 drops Frankincense and 2 drops Lavender
Toner: 3 drops Palmarosa and 2 drops Orange
Moisturiser: 2 drops Cedarwood and 3 drops Lavender
Bath/shower: 3 drops Lavender and 3 drops Palmarosa
Massage: 3 drops Rose and 2 drops Neroli

Combination skin
Cleanser: 3 drops Chamomile and 2 drops Ylang Ylang
Toner: 2 drops Juniperberry and 3 drops Geranium
Moisturiser: 2 drops Sandalwood and 3 drops Lavender
Bath/shower: 2 drops Myrtle and 4 drops Juniperberry
Massage: 2 drops Jasmine and 3 drops Geranium

Use the above recipes, but do experiment and try different combinations of oils. You may wish to stay with the same blend throughout your routine - just remember that you should regularly change your oils so that your body and sense of smell does not become immune to their benefits.

A skin condition not listed in Chapter 4, which can be very

effectively treated with Essential Oils, is stretch marks. These can be avoided if you use the recommended oils from four months into the pregnancy right through to just before the birth. Moisturiser, lotion, cream, bath and massage are all good methods to use. Our recommendations are Frankincense, Lavender, Mandarin, Neroli, and Orange. Use the oils individually or in a blend of two or three different oils. Scar tissue can be treated in the same way.

Hair care

Chapter 4 covers several hair problems, for example hair loss, dandruff and lice. Hair is made from the same material as nails - keratin - which is found in skin itself. The condition of their hair is very important to most people as it is so visible to the world. Hair condition is also a very good indication of the general state of your health. If there are any major changes in the condition of your hair it is quite likely that there is an underlying condition.

Essential Oils can be added to fragrance-free shampoos and conditioners and used in the same way as shop-bought products. There are many oils that can be used for different hair types. Rosemary has long been known for its affinity to hair and is used extensively in Aromatherapy for hair conditions. It is particularly useful for thinning hair or baldness.

Hair care Essential Oils by hair type
Dry and damaged
Chamomile; Geranium; Lavender; Myrrh; Orange; Sandalwood; Ylang Ylang

Greasy
Bergamot; Cedarwood; Eucalyptus; Geranium; Grapefruit; Juniperberry; Lavender; Lemon; Lemongrass; Rosemary; Spearmint; Tangerine; Tea Tree; Ylang Ylang

Normal
Chamomile; Lavender; Mandarin; Patchouli; Rosemary; Rosewood; Sandalwood

Dandruff
Cedarwood; Juniperberry; Lavender; Myrrh; Patchouli; Peppermint; Rosemary; Spearmint; Tea Tree

You can use the oils in both shampoos and conditioners in the same blends. The oils can also be used in massage carriers and then applied to the hair. One of the best carrier oils to use on the hair is Jojoba. Alternatively you can blend the Essential Oils, or use them individually, and put them on your hair during the last rinse.

Hair care Essential Oils by oil

	Dry	Greasy	Normal	Fair	Dark	Treated
BERGAMOT		●				
CEDARWOOD		●				
CHAMOMILE	●		●	●		
EUCALYPTUS		●				
GERANIUM	●	●			●	
GRAPEFRUIT		●				
JUNIPERBERRY		●				
LAVENDER	●	●	●			●
LEMON		●		●		
LEMONGRASS		●				
MANDARIN			●			
MYRRH	●					
ORANGE	●					●
PATCHOULI			●		●	
ROSEMARY		●	●		●	
ROSEWOOD			●		●	
SANDALWOOD	●		●			
SPEARMINT		●				
TANGERINE		●				

	Dry	Greasy	Normal	Fair	Dark	Treated
TEA TREE		●				
YLANG YLANG	●	●				

Recipes

Try the following blends in your hair care routine. Use 10 drops for every 25 ml of shampoo or conditioner:

Dry: 2 drops Orange, 4 drops Lavender and 4 drops Geranium

Greasy: 2 drops Lemon, 4 drops Cedarwood and 4 drops Bergamot

Normal: 6 drops Rosemary and 4 drops Lavender

Dandruff: 2 drops Tea Tree, 4 drops Rosemary and 4 drops Lavender

Rinses

If you want to enhance the colour of your hair and give it an extra depth and shine, you can use Essential Oils in a warm water rinse. For dark hair add 2 drops Rosemary, 1 drop Rosewood and 1 drop Geranium to 1 litre of water. Rinse your hair with the water, then wrap a towel around it and keep it on for 2 to 3 hours, or as long as possible. Wash off with fragrance-free shampoo. If your hair is fair you should use the same process but with 2 drops Chamomile and 1 drop Lemon.

Look after your skin and hair. Taking those extra few minutes every day to follow these simple body care routines will pay great dividends in terms of health, looks and feeling good.

Chapter 6

The Essential Oils

New Essential Oils are being discovered regularly. There are at least 300 Essential Oils now available, all with their own aromas, properties and uses. Most of these are not used regularly by Aromatherapists as they may be too expensive, difficult to obtain, not proven, difficult to use, or are too specific in their therapeutic value. Most Aromatherapists will work with between 30 to 40 oils. It is quite possible to treat successfully all conditions that respond to Essential Oils with this small range.

The following pages detail 44 of what we consider to be the most frequently used and useful oils. It is not of course an exhaustive list, and there will be some who will suggest that this oil should have been included or that oil is less useful than this, and so on!

This simply illustrates that Aromatherapy is very much a personal choice activity, which is more of an art than a science. People will choose oils not only on the basis of their therapeutic value but also because they enjoy their aroma and they have had success with particular oils in the past.

However, there is a large body of opinion within Aromatherapy about the therapeutic value of the 44 oils listed here. This means that they are well used, tried and tested, and you can have confidence in their listed uses and properties.

If you want to know about an oil not listed here please look it up in one of the other books detailed in the 'Further reading' section at the end of this book.

Always remember to check the quality of any oil before you use it (see 'Quality of oils' in Chapter 1), and you will find an extensive list of Conditions and Treatment Suggestions that should help you to decide what oil to use and how to use it.

The entries explained

Each oil is listed with the following details:

Latin name: This identifies the oil exactly. There are many different species of plant with the same common name (for example, there are over 700 species of Geranium and 300 varieties of Tea Tree), but only one species will produce the most therapeutically valuable oil. Always make sure that you buy an oil with the correct Latin name to be sure of using the correct one.

Plant: This simply describes the type of plant from which the oil is obtained, for example tree, herb, etc.

Part: The part of the plant from which the oil is obtained, for example flowering tops, leaves, etc.

Note: Essential Oils evaporate at different rates, and as they do so their aroma changes. The evaporation rates are grouped into three types: Base, Middle and Top. (See Chapter 3, 'Blending oils')

Intensity: Each oil has a particular 'strength' of aroma, and this intensity is measured as either 'Low' - subtle and gentle - 'Medium' - fresh and stimulating - and High - strong and penetrating. Intensity is different from Note (as strength is to stamina), but most Top Note oils will be High intensity.

Keyword: One word that sums up the character of the oil. This should be taken as a guide only.

Aroma: Three words that consistently appear in descriptions of the Essential Oils. Again this should be taken as a guide only as your olfactory senses will be as individual as you are. I know many people who find the aroma of Tea Tree very pleasant!

Precautions: For most oils there are some occasions or conditions in which the oil should be avoided or used with care. These precautions should be followed to ensure healthy use of the oils. For further general precautions regarding oils please see Chapter 10.

Parts of body: Each oil has an affinity with particular parts of the body. This list is not exhaustive but simply indicates the parts of the body most benefited by the oil.

Major properties: These are the medical terms for the main therapeutic properties of each oil:

Analgesic
Relieves pain
Bergamot; Black Pepper; Chamomile; Coriander; Eucalyptus; Geranium; Ginger; Lavender; Marjoram; Niaouli; Peppermint; Rosemary; Rosewood

Antacid
Combats acid in the body
Lemon

Antibiotic
Combats infection in the body
Tea Tree

Anticoagulant
Prevents blood from clotting
Geranium

Antidepressant
Helps to lift the mood
Basil; Bergamot; Chamomile; Clary Sage; Geranium; Grapefruit; Jasmine; Lavender; Lemongrass; Lime; Litsea Cubeba; Neroli; Orange; Patchouli; Petitgrain; Rose; Rosemary; Rosewood; Ylang Ylang

Anti-emetic
Reduces vomiting
Chamomile; Ginger

Anti-inflammatory
Reduces inflammation
Chamomile; Clary Sage; Fennel; Lavender; Myrrh; Patchouli; Peppermint; Rose; Sandalwood; Scots Pine

Antirheumatic
Helps to relieve rheumatism
Chamomile; Eucalyptus; Juniperberry; Lavender; Lemon; Niaouli; Rosemary

Antispasmodic
Relieves cramp
Basil; Bergamot; Black Pepper; Chamomile; Citronella; Clary Sage; Coriander; Fennel; Jasmine; Juniperberry; Lavender; Mandarin;

Marjoram; Neroli; Orange; Peppermint; Petitgrain; Rose; Rosemary; Sandalwood; Spearmint; Tangerine; Thyme; Vetiver

Antisudorific
Reduces sweating
Clary Sage

Antiviral
Controls the growth of viruses
Eucalyptus; Lavender; Lime; Palmarosa; Tea Tree

Aperitif
Encourages appetite
Black Pepper; Ginger; Grapefruit; Lime; Litsea Cubeba; Thyme

Astringent
Tightens tissues and reduces fluid loss
Cedarwood; Frankincense; Geranium; Juniperberry; Lemon; Lime; Myrrh; Myrtle; Patchouli; Peppermint; Rosemary; Sandalwood; Spearmint; Thyme

Bactericide
Kills bacteria
Black Pepper; Citronella; Coriander; Eucalyptus; Lavender; Lemon; Lemongrass; Lime; Litsea Cubeba; Myrtle; Neroli; Niaouli; Palmarosa; Rose; Rosewood; Tea Tree; Thyme

Carminative
Helps expel gas from the intestines
Basil; Bergamot; Black Pepper; Chamomile; Clary Sage; Coriander; Fennel; Frankincense; Ginger; Juniperberry; Lavender; Lemon; Lemongrass; Marjoram; Myrrh; Neroli; Orange; Peppermint; Rosemary; Sandalwood; Spearmint; Tangerine; Thyme

Cephalic
Clears the mind, stimulates mental activity
Basil; Grapefruit; Rosemary

Decongestant
Helps release of nasal mucous
Eucalyptus; Lavender; Niaouli; Peppermint; Scots Pine; Spearmint

Deodorant
Reduces odour
Bergamot; Citronella; Clary Sage; Eucalyptus; Geranium; Lavender; Lemongrass; Litsea Cubeba; Melissa; Neroli; Patchouli; Petitgrain; Rosewood; Scots Pine

Detoxicant
Helps cleanse the body of impurities
Fennel; Juniperberry; Lavender

Digestive
Aids digestion
Basil; Bergamot; Black Pepper; Chamomile; Clary Sage; Coriander; Frankincense; Lemongrass; Litsea Cubeba; Mandarin; Marjoram; Neroli; Orange; Rosemary; Spearmint

Disinfectant
Destroys germs
Grapefruit; Juniperberry; Lime; Scots Pine

Diuretic
Increases production of urine
Black Pepper; Cedarwood; Chamomile; Citronella; Eucalyptus; Fennel; Frankincense; Geranium; Grapefruit; Juniperberry; Lavender; Lemon; Lemongrass; Patchouli; Rose; Rosemary; Sandalwood; Scots Pine; Spearmint; Tangerine; Thyme

Emetic
Induces vomiting
Rose

Emmenagogue
Encourages menstruation
Basil; Chamomile; Citronella; Clary Sage; Fennel; Juniperberry; Lavender; Marjoram; Peppermint; Rose; Rosemary; Spearmint, Thyme

Emollient
Soothes and softens the skin
Cedarwood; Chamomile; Jasmine; Lemon; Mandarin; Neroli; Sandalwood; Tangerine

Expectorant
Helps with expulsion of phlegm
Basil; Bergamot; Cedarwood; Eucalyptus; Fennel; Ginger; Marjoram; Myrrh; Myrtle; Peppermint; Sandalwood; Scots Pine; Spearmint; Tea Tree; Thyme

Febrifuge
Reduces fever
Basil; Bergamot; Black Pepper; Chamomile; Citronella; Eucalyptus; Ginger; Lemon; Lime; Niaouli; Orange; Palmarosa; Patchouli; Peppermint; Spearmint

Fungicide
Inhibits growth of fugal infection
Cedarwood; Citronella; Coriander; Lavender; Lemongrass; Melissa; Myrrh; Patchouli; Tea Tree; Thyme

Haemostatic
Arrests bleeding/haemorrhage
Geranium; Lemon; Lime; Rose

Hepatic
Strengthens the liver and gall bladder
Chamomile; Lemon; Peppermint; Rose; Rosemary; Spearmint

Hypertensive
Increases blood pressure
Rosemary; Thyme

Hypoglycaemiant
Lowers blood sugar
Eucalyptus; Geranium; Lemon

Hypotensive
Lowers blood pressure
Lavender; Lemon; Marjoram; Ylang Ylang

Insecticide
Kills insect pests
Cedarwood; Citronella; Eucalyptus; Fennel; Geranium; Juniperberry; Lemon; Lemongrass; Lime; Litsea Cubeba; Niaouli; Patchouli; Rosewood; Tea Tree

Nervine
Strengthens the nervous system
Basil; Chamomile; Clary Sage; Juniperberry; Lavender; Marjoram;
Peppermint; Rosemary; Spearmint; Thyme

Rubefacient
Produces warmth and redness
Black Pepper, Citronella; Eucalyptus; Ginger; Juniperberry; Scots
Pine; Thyme; Vetiver

Sedative
Calms the nervous system
Bergamot; Cedarwood; Chamomile; Clary Sage; Frankincense;
Jasmine; Lavender; Mandarin; Marjoram; Myrrh; Myrtle; Neroli;
Orange; Patchouli; Petitgrain; Rose; Sandalwood; Vetiver; Ylang Ylang

Stimulant
Increases the flow of adrenaline and energy
Basil; Black Pepper; Coriander; Eucalyptus; Fennel; Ginger;
Grapefruit; Juniperberry; Lemongrass; Litsea Cubeba; Niaouli;
Peppermint; Rosemary; Rosewood; Scots Pine; Spearmint;
Tangerine; Tea Tree; Thyme; Vetiver

Styptic
Arrests external bleeding
Geranium; Lemon

Sudorific
Increases perspiration
Chamomile; Fennel; Ginger; Juniperberry; Lavender; Peppermint;
Rosemary; Scots Pine; Tea Tree; Thyme

Uterine
Acts as a tonic for the womb
Clary Sage; Frankincense; Jasmine; Myrrh

Vasoconstrictor
Contracts the blood vessels
Geranium; Peppermint

Vasodilator
Expands the blood vessels
Marjoram

Vulnerary
Helps wounds to heal
Bergamot; Chamomile; Eucalyptus; Frankincense; Geranium; Juniperberry; Lavender; Litsea Cubeba; Marjoram; Myrrh; Niaouli; Rosemary

Blends: Lists all the other oils that are consistently talked about as very good blends with this particular oil. Remember though that it is all a matter of taste - follow the rules (see Chapter 3, 'Blending oils') and experiment to find the blend that suits you.

Alphabetical list of 44 Essential Oils

BASIL
Ocimum basilicum

Plant: herb	*Part:* flowering heads and leaves
Note: top	*Intensity:* medium
Keyword: cooling	*Aroma:* spicy; sweet

Precautions: avoid during pregnancy and with epilepsy; may irritate sensitive skin
Parts of body: respiration; digestion; immune system; mind; circulation; muscles; genito-urinary
Major properties: antidepressant; antispasmodic; carminative; cephalic; digestive; emmenagogue; expectorant; febrifuge; nervine; stimulant (of the adrenal cortex)
Blends: Bergamot; Clary Sage; Coriander; Lime; Citronella; Geranium; Lavender; Myrrh; Spearmint; Vetiver; Tangerine; Thyme

BERGAMOT
Citrus bergamia

Plant: tree	*Part:* peel of fruit
Note: top	*Intensity:* low
Keyword: refreshing	*Aroma:* fresh; light; citrus

Precautions: do not use in sunlight; may irritate some sensitive skins
Parts of body: urinary tract; digestion; respiration; skin; mind
Major properties: analgesic; antidepressant; antispasmodic; carminative; deodorant; digestive; expectorant; febrifuge; sedative; vulnerary
Blends: Basil; Black Pepper; Cedarwood; Chamomile; Citronella; Eucalyptus; Geranium; Juniperberry; Lavender; Lemon; Lime; Mandarin; Marjoram; Myrtle; Neroli; Palmarosa; Patchouli; Petitgrain; Thyme; Ylang Ylang

BLACK PEPPER

Piper nigrum

Plant: shrub	*Part:* fruit
Note: middle	*Intensity:* high
Keywords: penetrating/stimulating	*Aroma:* warm; sharp; spicy

Precautions: reduce quantities for sensitive skin

Parts of body: muscles; joints; digestion; circulation; respiratory

Major properties: analgesic; antispasmodic; aperitif; bactericide; carminative; digestive; diuretic; febrifuge; rubefacient; stimulant

Blends: Bergamot; Frankincense; Geranium; Ginger; Grapefruit; Lavender; Lemon; Mandarin; Myrtle; Orange; Rosemary; Sandalwood; Ylang Ylang

CEDARWOOD

Cedrus atlantica

Plant: tree	*Part:* wood
Note: base	*Intensity:* low
Keyword: calming	*Aroma:* soft; woody; smoky

Precautions: avoid in pregnancy

Parts of body: respiration; urinary tract; kidneys; muscles; mind

Major properties: astringent; diuretic; emollient; expectorant; fungicide; insecticide; sedative

Blends: Bergamot; Citronella; Clary Sage; Frankincense; Geranium; Grapefruit; Jasmine; Juniperberry; Lavender; Lemon; Lemongrass; Litsea Cubeba; Mandarin; Myrtle; Neroli; Peppermint; Petitgrain; Rose; Rosemary; Scots Pine

CHAMOMILE (ROMAN)

Anthemis nobilis

Plant: herb	*Part:* flowers
Note: middle	*Intensity:* high
Keyword: soothing	*Aroma:* fruity; apple-like; herby

Precautions: avoid with heavy periods, and in early pregnancy

Parts of body: muscles; head; nerves; genito-urinary; digestion; blood; skin; mind

Major properties: analgesic; antidepressant; anti-emetic; anti-inflammatory; antirheumatic; antispasmodic; carminative; digestive; diuretic; emmenagogue; emollient; febrifuge; hepatic; nervine; sedative; sudorific; vulnerary

Blends: Basil; Bergamot; Geranium; Grapefruit; Jasmine; Lavender; Lemon; Litsea Cubeba; Mandarin; Marjoram; Neroli; Palmarosa; Patchouli; Rose; Tangerine; Thyme; Ylang Ylang

CITRONELLA

Cymbopogon nardus

Plant: grass   *Part:* leaves/all parts
Note: top   *Intensity:* high
Keyword: refreshing   *Aroma:* lemony; powerful

Precautions: avoid during pregnancy; may irritate sensitive skin

Parts of body: nerves; skin; immune system; digestion; joints; mind

Major properties: antispasmodic; bactericide; deodorant; diuretic; emmenagogue; febrifuge; fungicide; insecticide; rubefacient

Blends: Basil; Bergamot; Cedarwood; Eucalyptus; Lemongrass; Melissa; Rosemary; Scots Pine; Tea Tree

CLARY SAGE

Salvia sclarea

Plant: herb   *Part:* flowering tops and foliage
Note: middle/top   *Intensity:* low
Keyword: euphoric   *Aroma:* nutty; warm; heavy

Precautions: avoid if driving, with alcohol and in pregnancy

Parts of body: hormones; genito-urinary; digestion; muscles; mind

Major properties: antidepressant; anti-inflammatory; antispasmodic; antisudorific; carminative; deodorant; digestive; emmenagogue; nervine; sedative; uterine

Blends: Basil; Bergamot; Cedarwood; Frankincense; Geranium; Jasmine; Juniperberry; Lavender; Lime; Patchouli; Sandalwood; Vetiver

CORIANDER

Coriandrum sativum

Plant: herb   *Part:* plant
Note: top   *Intensity:* medium/high
Keyword: stimulating   *Aroma:* herby; green; spicy

Precautions: use in moderation

Parts of body: circulation; muscles; joints; digestive; immune system; nerves

Major properties: analgesic; antirheumatic; antispasmodic; aphrodisiac; bactericide; carminative; digestive; fungicide; stimulant

Blends: Basil; Geranium; Lavender; Lemon; Marjoram; Rosemary; Vetiver

EUCALYPTUS

Eucalyptus globulus

Plant: tree   *Part:* leaves
Note: top   *Intensity:* high
Keyword: penetrating   *Aroma:* refreshing; sharp;
                                                    piercing

Precautions: avoid with epilepsy or diabetes

Parts of body: respiration; genito-urinary; muscles; nerves; skin; mind
Major properties: analgesic; antirheumatic; antiviral; bactericide; decongestant; deodorant; diuretic; expectorant; febrifuge;
hypoglycaemiant; insecticide; rubefacient; stimulant; vulnerary
Blends: Bergamot; Citronella; Ginger; Juniperberry; Lavender; Lemon; Lemongrass; Litsea Cubeba; Myrtle; Scots Pine; Spearmint; Tea Tree; Thyme

FENNEL (SWEET)
Foeniculum vulgare

Plant: herb	*Part:* seeds
Note: middle/top	*Intensity:* medium
Keyword: balancing	*Aroma:* aniseed; herby; spicy

Precautions: avoid during pregnancy and with epilepsy; may irritate sensitive skin
Parts of body: digestion; kidneys; respiration; hormones; genito-urinary; skin; mind
Major properties: anti-inflammatory; antispasmodic; carminative; detoxicant; diuretic; emmenagogue; expectorant; insecticide; stimulant; sudorific
Blends: Geranium; Lavender; Lemon; Melissa; Niaouli; Rose; Rosemary; Sandalwood

FRANKINCENSE
Boswellia Carteri/thurifera

Plant: tree	*Part:* bark/resin
Note: base/middle	*Intensity:* medium
Keyword: inspiring	*Aroma:* lemony; spicy; warm

Precautions: none
Parts of body: respiration; genito-urinary; digestion
Major properties: astringent; carminative; digestive; diuretic; sedative; uterine; vulnerary
Blends: Black Pepper; Cedarwood; Clary Sage; Geranium; Ginger; Grapefruit; Juniperberry; Lavender; Lemon; Myrrh; Orange; Patchouli; Rosemary; Rosewood; Sandalwood; Scots Pine

GERANIUM
Pelargonium graveolens

Plant: herb/plant	*Part:* flowers and leaves
Note: middle	*Intensity:* medium
Keyword: balancing	*Aroma:* sweet; floral; rose-like

Precautions: avoid during pregnancy or if you suffer from diabetes
Parts of body: hormones; genito-urinary; digestion; kidneys; circulation; respiration; nerves; skin; mind
Major properties: analgesic; anticoagulant; antidepressant; astringent; deodorant; diuretic; haemostatic; hypoglycaemiant; insecticide; styptic; vasoconstrictor; vulnerary

Blends: Bergamot; Black Pepper; Cedarwood; Chamomile; Clary Sage; Coriander; Fennel; Frankincense; Ginger; Grapefruit; Jasmine; Juniperberry; Lavender; Lime; Litsea Cubeba; Myrrh; Myrtle; Neroli; Orange; Palmarosa; Patchouli; Petitgrain; Rose; Rosemary; Rosewood; Sandalwood; Vetiver

GINGER

Zingiber officinale

Plant: herb	*Part:* root
Note: top	*Intensity:* high
Keyword: warming	*Aroma:* warm; spicy; sharp

Precautions: reduce dosage if it irritates sensitive skins

Parts of body: respiration; digestion; muscles; circulation; skin; mind

Major properties: analgesic; anti-emetic; aperitif; carminative; expectorant; febrifuge; rubefacient; stimulant; sudorific

Blends: Basil; Black Pepper; Eucalyptus; Frankincense; Geranium; Lemon; Lime; Litsea Cubeba; Orange; Patchouli; Rosemary; Tea Tree; Vetiver

GRAPEFRUIT

Citrus paradisi

Plant: tree	*Part:* peel of fruit
Note: top	*Intensity:* high
Keyword: uplifting	*Aroma:* tangy; sweet; refreshing

Precautions: do not use in sunlight; may irritate sensitive skin

Parts of body: digestion; kidneys; head; mind

Major properties: antidepressant; aperitif; cephalic; disinfectant; diuretic; stimulant

Blends: Bergamot; Black Pepper; Cedarwood; Chamomile; Frankincense; Geranium; Jasmine; Juniperberry; Lavender; Litsea Cubeba; Mandarin; Melissa; Palmarosa; Rose; Rosemary; Rosewood; Ylang Ylang

JASMINE

Jasminum officinale

Plant: tree	*Part:* flowers
Note: base	*Intensity:* medium
Keyword: exotic	*Aroma:* heady; flowery; sweet

Precautions: avoid in pregnancy (use at birth); reduce dosage

Parts of body: hormones; genito-urinary; respiration; muscles; skin; mind

Major properties: antidepressant; antispasmodic; emollient; sedative; uterine

Blends: Bergamot; Eucalyptus; Frankincense; Geranium; Mandarin; Neroli; Orange; Palmarosa; Rose; Rosewood; Sandalwood; Spearmint; Vetiver

JUNIPERBERRY
Juniperus communis

Plant: bush	*Part:* berries
Note: middle	*Intensity:* low
Keyword: cleansing	*Aroma:* refreshing; herby; woody

Precautions: avoid with kidney disease and during pregnancy

Parts of body: genito-urinary; kidneys; digestion; muscles; nerves; skin; mind

Major properties: antirheumatic; antispasmodic; astringent; carminative; detoxicant; disinfectant; diuretic; emmenagogue; insecticide; nervine; rubefacient; stimulant; sudorific; vulnerary

Blends: Bergamot; Cedarwood; Clary Sage; Frankincense; Geranium; Grapefruit; Lemon; Lemongrass; Lime; Myrrh; Niaouli; Orange; Rosemary; Sandalwood

LAVENDER
Lavendula officinalis/angustifolium

Plant: shrub	*Part:* flowers
Note: middle	*Intensity:* low
Keyword: soothing	*Aroma:* floral; light; woody

Precautions: avoid in early stages of pregnancy

Parts of body: circulation; muscles; respiration; genito-urinary; kidneys; digestion; nerves; skin; mind

Major properties: analgesic; antidepressant; anti-inflammatory; antirheumatic; antispasmodic; antiviral; bactericide; carminative; decongestant; deodorant; detoxicant; diuretic; emmenagogue; fungicide; hypotensive; nervine; sedative; sudorific; vulnerary

Blends: Basil; Bergamot; Black Pepper; Cedarwood; Chamomile; Citronella; Clary Sage; Coriander; Eucalyptus; Fennel; Frankincense; Geranium; Ginger; Grapefruit; Jasmine; Juniperberry; Lemon; Lemongrass; Lime; Litsea Cubeba; Mandarin; Marjoram; Melissa; Myrrh; Myrtle; Neroli; Niaouli; Orange; Palmarosa; Patchouli; Peppermint; Petitgrain; Rose; Rosemary; Rosewood; Sandalwood; Scots Pine; Spearmint; Tangerine; Tea Tree; Thyme; Vetiver; Ylang Ylang

LEMON
Citrus limonum

Plant: tree	*Part:* peel of fruit
Note: top	*Intensity:* high
Keyword: refreshing	*Aroma:* fresh; strong; sharp

Precautions: avoid in sunlight; may irritate sensitive skin, avoid if diabetic

Parts of body: circulation; respiration; digestion; kidneys; head; nerves; muscles; skin

Major properties: antacid; antirheumatic; astringent; bactericide; carminative; diuretic; emollient; febrifuge; haemostatic; hepatic; hypoglycaemiant; hypotensive; insecticide; styptic

Blends: Black Pepper; Bergamot; Cedarwood; Chamomile; Clary Sage; Coriander; Eucalyptus; Fennel; Frankincense; Ginger; Juniperberry; Lavender; Mandarin; Melissa; Myrtle; Niaouli; Neroli; Rose; Sandalwood; Tea Tree; Thyme; Ylang Ylang

LEMONGRASS

Cymbopogon citratus

Plant: grass	*Part:* leaves
Note: top	*Intensity:* high
Keyword: tonic	*Aroma:* fresh; strong; sweet

Precautions: may irritate sensitive skin; reduce dosage

Parts of body: nerves; digestion; respiration; muscles; circulation; head; skin; mind

Major properties: antidepressant; bactericide; carminative; deodorant; digestive; diuretic; fungicide; insecticide; stimulant

Blends: Cedarwood; Citronella; Eucalyptus; Geranium; Jasmine; Juniperberry; Lavender; Melissa; Myrrh; Neroli; Niaouli; Palmarosa; Patchouli; Rosemary; Tea Tree

LIME

Citrus aurantifolia/medica

Plant: tree	*Part:* peel of fruit
Note: top	*Intensity:* high
Keyword: stimulating	*Aroma:* sharp; bright; bitter-sweet

Precautions: do not use in sunlight; may irritate sensitive skin

Parts of body: respiration; digestion; muscles; skin; mind

Major properties: antidepressant; antiviral; aperitif; astringent; bactericide; disinfectant; febrifuge; haemostatic; insecticide

Blends: Basil; Bergamot; Clary Sage; Geranium; Ginger; Juniperberry; Lavender; Mandarin; Melissa; Neroli; Niaouli; Palmarosa; Rose; Rosemary; Ylang Ylang

LITSEA CUBEBA

Litsea citrata

Plant: tree	*Part:* fruit
Note: top	*Intensity:* medium
Keyword: refreshing	*Aroma:* sweet; fresh; fruity

Precautions: none

Parts of body: circulation; digestive; immune; mind; skin

Major properties: antidepressant; aperitif; bactericide; deodorant; digestive; insecticide; stimulant; vulnerary

Blends: Cedarwood; Chamomile; Eucalyptus; Geranium; Ginger; Grapefruit; Palmarosa; Patchouli; Tea Tree; Ylang Ylang

MANDARIN

Citrus madurensis/nobilis

Plant: tree

Note: top/middle

Keyword: revitalising

Part: peel of fruit

Intensity: medium

Aroma: delicate; sweet; tangy

Precautions: do not use in sunlight

Parts of body: digestion; liver; skin; mind

Major properties: antispasmodic; digestive; emollient; sedative

Blends: Bergamot; Black Pepper; Chamomile; Grapefruit; Lavender; Lemon; Lime; Marjoram; Melissa; Myrtle; Neroli; Palmarosa; Peppermint; Petitgrain; Rose; Rosemary; Tea Tree

MARJORAM

Origanum marjorana

Plant: herb

Note: middle

Keyword: relaxing

Part: flowering heads and leaves

Intensity: low

Aroma: warm; penetrating; peppery

Precautions: avoid during pregnancy

Parts of body: muscles; circulation; head; digestion; respiration; genito-urinary; skin; mind

Major properties: analgesic; antispasmodic; carminative; digestive; emmenagogue; expectorant; hypotensive; nervine; sedative; vasodilator; vulnerary

Blends: Bergamot; Cedarwood; Chamomile; Coriander; Lavender; Mandarin; Orange; Peppermint; Rosemary; Rosewood; Tangerine; Vetiver; Ylang Ylang

MELISSA

Melissa officinalis

Plant: herb

Note: middle

Keyword: refreshing

Part: leaves

Intensity: high

Aroma: fresh; lemony; light

Precautions: none

Parts of body: mind; skin; digestion

Major properties: deodorant; fungicide

Blends: Bergamot; Cedarwood; Citronella; Fennel; Grapefruit; Lemon; Lemongrass; Lime; Mandarin; Orange; Vetiver

MYRRH

Commiphora myrrha

Plant: tree

Note: base

Keyword: healing

Part: bark/resin

Intensity: medium

Aroma: musty; bitter; earthy

Precautions: should not be used during pregnancy

Parts of body: digestion; genito-urinary; mind; respiration; skin
Major properties: anti-inflammatory; astringent; carminative; expectorant; fungicide; sedative; uterine; vulnerary
Blends: Basil; Eucalyptus; Frankincense; Geranium; Juniperberry; Lavender; Lemongrass; Palmarosa; Patchouli; Sandalwood; Tea Tree

MYRTLE

Myrtus communis

Plant: bush	*Part:* leaves, twigs and flowers
Note: middle/base	*Intensity:* medium
Keyword: gentle	*Aroma:* fresh, clear, herby
Precautions: none	

Parts of body: skin, respiration, immune system
Major properties: antiseptic, astringent, bactericide, expectorant, sedative
Blends: Bergamot; Black Pepper; Cedarwood; Eucalyptus; Geranium; Lavender; Lemon; Mandarin; Orange; Patchouli; Petitgrain; Rosemary; Sandalwood; Scots Pine; Tea Tree; Ylang Ylang

NEROLI

Citrus aurantium/vulgaris

Plant: tree	*Part:* petals
Note: middle/base	*Intensity:* low
Keyword: relaxing	*Aroma:* floral; bitter-sweet; distinctive
Precautions: none	

Parts of body: nerves; head; digestion; circulation; skin; mind
Major properties: antidepressant; antispasmodic; bactericide; carminative; deodorant; digestive; emollient; sedative
Blends: Bergamot; Geranium; Jasmine; Lavender; Lemon; Lime; Orange; Palmarosa; Petitgrain; Rose; Rosemary; Sandalwood; Tangerine; Ylang Ylang

NIAOULI

Melaleuca viridiflora

Plant: tree	*Part:* leaves and young twigs
Note: top	*Intensity:* high
Keyword: penetrating	*Aroma:* strong; hot; sweet
Precautions: none	

Parts of body: digestion; genito-urinary; head; respiration; skin; mind
Major properties: analgesic; antirheumatic; bactericide; decongestant; febrifuge; insecticide; stimulant; vulnerary
Blends: Fennel; Juniperberry; Lavender; Lemon; Lemongrass; Lime; Orange; Patchouli; Peppermint; Rosemary; Scots Pine

ORANGE

Citrus sinensis

Plant: tree   *Part:* peel of fruit
Note: top   *Intensity:* high
Keyword: cheering   *Aroma:* zesty; sweet; refreshing
Precautions: avoid in sunlight and may irritate sensitive skin
Parts of body: digestion; respiration; muscles; skin; mind
Major properties: antidepressant; antispasmodic; carminative; digestive; febrifuge; sedative
Blends: Black Pepper; Frankincense; Geranium; Ginger; Jasmine; Juniperberry; Lavender; Marjoram; Melissa; Myrtle; Neroli; Niaouli; Palmarosa; Petitgrain; Rose; Rosewood; Tea Tree; Vetiver; Ylang Ylang

PALMAROSA

Cymbopogon martini

Plant: grass   *Part:* leaves
Note: top   *Intensity:* medium
Keyword: calming   *Aroma:* sweet; floral; rose-like
Precautions: none
Parts of body: digestion; skin; mind
Major properties: antiviral; bactericide; febrifuge
Blends: Bergamot; Black Pepper; Chamomile; Geranium; Grapefruit; Jasmine; Lavender; Lemongrass; Lime; Litsea Cubeba; Mandarin; Myrrh; Orange; Petitgrain; Rose; Rosewood; Sandalwood; Tangerine; Ylang Ylang

PATCHOULI

Pogostemon patchouli

Plant: shrub   *Part:* leaves
Note: base   *Intensity:* high
Keyword: penetrating   *Aroma:* musky; sweet; earthy
Precautions: reduce dosage as aroma lingers
Parts of body: skin; digestion; mind
Major properties: antidepressant; anti-inflammatory; astringent; deodorant; diuretic; febrifuge; fungicide; insecticide; sedative
Blends: Bergamot; Chamomile; Clary Sage; Frankincense; Geranium; Ginger; Lavender; Lemongrass; Litsea Cubeba; Myrrh; Myrtle; Neroli; Niaouli; Rosewood; Sandalwood; Scots Pine; Vetiver; Ylang Ylang

PEPPERMINT

Mentha piperita

Plant: herb

Part: leaves and flowering tops

Note: top/middle

Intensity: medium

Keyword: cooling

Aroma: menthol; sharp; piercing

Precautions: avoid during pregnancy and when nursing babies; may irritate sensitive skin

Parts of body: digestion; head; genito-urinary; nerves; respiration; skin; mind

Major properties: analgesic; anti-inflammatory; antispasmodic; astringent; carminative; decongestant; emmenagogue; expectorant; febrifuge; hepatic; nervine; stimulant; sudorific; vasoconstrictor

Blends: Cedarwood; Lavender; Mandarin; Marjoram; Niaouli; Rosemary; Scots Pine; Spearmint

PETITGRAIN

Citrus aurantium bigaradia

Plant: tree

Part: leaves and young twigs

Note: middle/top

Intensity: low

Keyword: refreshing

Aroma: woody; floral; light

Precautions: none

Parts of body: nerves; skin; mind

Major properties: antidepressant; antispasmodic; deodorant; sedative

Blends: Bergamot; Cedarwood; Geranium; Lavender; Mandarin; Myrtle; Neroli; Orange; Palmarosa; Rosemary; Rosewood; Sandalwood; Tangerine; Ylang Ylang

ROSE

Rosa damascena

Plant: flower

Part: petals

Note: middle/base

Intensity: high

Keyword: cleansing

Aroma: deep; sweet; floral

Precautions: avoid in early pregnancy

Parts of body: genito-urinary; circulation; digestion; head; respiration; skin; mind

Major properties: antidepressant; anti-inflammatory; antispasmodic; bactericide; diuretic; emetic; emmenagogue; haemostatic; hepatic; sedative

Blends: Bergamot; Chamomile; Clary Sage; Geranium; Jasmine; Lavender; Neroli; Orange; Palmarosa; Patchouli; Sandalwood

ROSEMARY

Rosmarinus officinalis

Plant: herb

Part: flowering tops and leaves

Note: middle

Intensity: high

Keyword: stimulating

Aroma: strong; herbal; refreshing

Precautions: avoid with high blood pressure and during pregnancy; use minimum dosage with epilepsy
Parts of body: circulation; digestion; genito-urinary; head; muscles; nerves; respiration; skin; mind
Major properties: analgesic; antidepressant; antirheumatic; antispasmodic; astringent; carminative; cephalic; digestive; diuretic; emmenagogue; hepatic; hypertensive; nervine; stimulant; sudorific; vulnerary
Blends: Black Pepper; Cedarwood; Citronella; Coriander; Fennel; Frankincense; Geranium; Ginger; Grapefruit; Juniperberry; Lavender; Lemongrass; Lime; Mandarin; Marjoram; Myrtle; Niaouli; Orange; Peppermint; Petitgrain; Rosewood; Scots Pine; Spearmint; Tea Tree

ROSEWOOD

Aniba roseaodora
Plant: tree
Note: middle/top
Keyword: tonic
Part: wood
Intensity: medium
Aroma: floral; spicy; sweet
Precautions: none
Parts of body: respiration; head; skin; mind
Major properties: analgesic; antidepressant; bactericide; deodorant; insecticide; stimulant
Blends: Cedarwood; Frankincense; Geranium; Grapefruit; Lavender; Marjoram; Orange; Palmarosa; Patchouli; Petitgrain; Rose; Rosemary; Sandalwood; Ylang Ylang

SANDALWOOD

Santalum album
Plant: tree
Note: base
Keyword: calming
Part: heartwood
Intensity: low
Aroma: subtle; rich; sweet
Precautions: reduce dosage as aroma lingers
Parts of body: genito-urinary; kidneys; respiration; digestion; skin; mind
Major properties: anti-inflammatory; antispasmodic; astringent; carminative; diuretic; emollient; expectorant; sedative
Blends: Black Pepper; Clary Sage; Fennel; Frankincense; Geranium; Jasmine; Juniperberry; Lavender; Lemon; Myrrh; Myrtle; Neroli; Palmarosa; Patchouli; Petitgrain; Rose; Rosewood; Vetiver; Ylang Ylang

SCOTS PINE

Pinus sylvestris
Plant: tree
Note: middle
Keyword: strengthening
Part: needles and cones
Intensity: high
Aroma: pine; fresh; resinous

Precautions: reduce dosage if it irritates sensitive skin
Parts of body: respiration; kidneys; circulation; muscles; digestion; skin; mind
Major properties: anti-inflammatory; decongestant; deodorant; disinfectant; diuretic; expectorant; rubefacient; stimulant; sudorific
Blends: Cedarwood; Citronella; Eucalyptus; Frankincense; Geranium; Lavender; Myrtle; Niaouli; Patchouli; Peppermint; Rosemary; Tea Tree

SPEARMINT

Mentha spicata

Plant: herb	*Part:* leaves, flowering tops
Note: top	*Intensity:* medium
Keyword: calming	*Aroma:* fresh mild mint

Precautions: avoid during pregnancy
Parts of body: digestion; mind; respiration; nerves; skin; immune system
Major properties: antispasmodic; astringent; carminative; decongestive; digestive; diuretic; emmenagogue; expectorant; febrifuge; hepatic; nervine; stimulant
Blends: Basil; Eucalyptus; Geranium; Jasmine; Lavender; Peppermint; Rosemary; Tangerine; Tea Tree; Vetiver

TANGERINE

Citrus madurensis

Plant: tree	*Part:* peel of fruit
Note: top/middle	*Intensity:* medium
Keyword: arousing	*Aroma:* fine, sweet orange

Precautions: do not use in sunlight
Parts of body: skin; muscles; circulation; nerves; digestion; mind
Major properties: antispasmodic; carminative; diuretic; stimulant
Blends: Basil; Chamomile, Lavender; Marjoram; Neroli; Palmarosa; Petitgrain; Spearmint

TEA TREE

Melaleuca alternifolia

Plant: tree/bush	*Part:* leaves and twigs
Note: top	*Intensity:* high
Keyword: cleansing	*Aroma:* medicinal; sanitary; pungent

Precautions: may irritate sensitive skin
Parts of body: circulation; genito-urinary; muscles; respiration; skin
Major properties: antibiotic; antiviral; bactericide; expectorant; fungicide; insecticide; stimulant; sudorific
Blends: Citronella; Eucalyptus; Ginger; Lavender; Lemon; Lemongrass; Litsea Cubeba; Mandarin; Myrrh; Myrtle; Orange; Rosemary; Scots Pine; Spearmint

THYME (GENTLE)

Thymus vulgaris linalool

Plant: herb   *Part:* plant
Note: middle   *Intensity:* medium
Keyword: balancing   *Aroma:* warm, herby
Precautions: none

Parts of body: skin; muscles; joints; circulation; respiration; digestive; genito-urinary; nerves

Major properties: antispasmodic; aperitif; astringent; bactericide; carminative; diuretic; emmenagogue; expectorant; fungicide; hypertensive; nervine; rubefacient; stimulant

Blends: Basil; Bergamot; Chamomile; Eucalyptus; Geranium; Lavender; Lemon

VETIVER

Vetiveria zizanoides

Plant: grass   *Part:* roots
Note: base   *Intensity:* low
Keyword: tranquillity   *Aroma:* smoky; earthy; woody
Precautions: avoid during pregnancy

Parts of body: skin; muscles; circulation; nerves; joints

Major properties: antispasmodic; rubefacient; sedative (nerves); stimulant (circulation)

Blends: Basil; Clary Sage; Coriander; Ginger; Jasmine; Lavender; Marjoram; Melissa; Orange; Patchouli; Sandalwood; Spearmint; Ylang Ylang;

YLANG YLANG

Cananga odorata

Plant: tree   *Part:* flowers
Note: base   *Intensity:* medium
Keyword: soothing   *Aroma:* heavy; sweet; floral
Precautions: may cause headaches/nausea if over-used; avoid on inflammatory skin conditions

Parts of body: hormones; genito-urinary; nerves; skin; mind

Major properties: antidepressant; hypotensive; sedative

Blends: Bergamot; Black Pepper; Chamomile; Grapefruit; Jasmine; Lavender; Lemon; Lime; Litsea Cubeba; Marjoram; Myrtle; Neroli; Orange; Palmarosa; Patchouli; Petitgrain; Rose; Rosewood; Sandalwood; Vetiver

Chapter 7

Aromatherapy
around the house

M ost people think of Aromatherapy as a form of treatment and confine its use to those times when we are feeling a little under the weather. However, there are far wider uses for Essential Oils and in this chapter we will take a look at some of the ways in which you can use them in and around your home, not only in creating a pleasant atmosphere, but also in some practical applications.

Take a look at the labels on your household products and see how many Essential Oils are used to clean and care for your home. You cannot watch the television without seeing or hearing about the natural powers of oils being harnessed in the commonest of branded products, including candles, cleaners and a host of others. Now is the time to be protective and allow your house to be part of the prevention of illness rather than a home in which to recover.

Essential Oils around your home do more than just get rid of unpleasant odours and soften bad tempers. Many oils have powerful properties that destroy bacteria more effectively than many household cleaners. They are true natural cleaning agents and do not harm the balance of nature in the process. The hole in the ozone layer will get no bigger if we draw on the strength of the natural, pure cleaning power of Essential Oils!

Creating an ambience

There are many factors to consider when making your house into a home, from the colour of the walls to the type of lighting, heating, furnishings and belongings that we gather around us. Each home is unique to its occupants and our taste will be reflected in our surroundings. We pay a great deal of attention to what we can *see* around the home; we surround ourselves with marvellous textures in our wallcoverings, upholstery and ornaments. Our ears are filled with the sound of our favourite music played on our increasingly complex music systems. Our senses are bombarded with a barrage of stimulation. Yet the one sense that seems to be so often forgotten is our sense of smell. We just cannot resist going up to a vase of flowers to enjoy the bouquet. Nice smells make us feel good, and we could all do with a little more of the 'feel-good factor' in our lives!

Whatever kind of home you have, Essential Oils can make the difference to the way it is perceived by both you and your guests. Let us not forget that unlike the fixtures and fittings, which are both costly and time-consuming to change, an aroma can be adjusted within minutes to suit your mood, and it will not require a re-mortgage to pay for it! In a recent report by estate agents it was suggested that house sales were increased when the aroma of coffee or a citrus oil were present during viewing. It appears that the fragrance made the properties more appealing, and the sales of houses not only increased, but the time of the sale was also reduced by a quarter of the original completion time.

You can bring a clean fresh fragrance to any room of your home by using any of the methods listed in this book. You may wish to use an aroma to welcome you and your guests as you enter your home by using Essential Oils in your reception rooms, or you may wish to concentrate on the trouble spots around the house like the laundry basket, drains, shed, garage or greenhouse.

Below are a few suggested oils that you could use to match the mood of the occasion in your home. They can be used in a room burner, made into room sprays, used in humidifiers, or in any of the other ways listed in this chapter to create the desired affect. If you wish to mix together Essential Oils to create your own fragrance, we suggest that you use no more than four oils in each blend. Getting the right balance without an individual aroma masking the other fragrances may take more than one attempt, but it is well worth trying your own combination.

Balancing
Clary Sage; Geranium; Jasmine; Lemon; Melissa; Palmarosa

Calming
Clary Sage; Fennel; Frankincense; Ginger; Marjoram; Orange

Refreshing
Bergamot; Eucalyptus; Litsea Cubeba; Peppermint; Spearmint; Tangerine

Relaxing
Cedarwood; Chamomile; Jasmine; Myrrh; Neroli; Rose; Vetiver

Revitalising
Bergamot; Citronella; Eucalyptus; Lemon; Lime

Sensual
Basil; Patchouli; Rose; Sandalwood; Ylang Ylang

Candles

Candle-making can be an inexpensive hobby and can also be great fun. It is possible to mix small quantities of both Essential Oils and refresher oils into molten wax before the candle is made, *but remember that caution should always be taken when dealing with hot or flammable liquid.*

It is important not to add too much Essential Oil or the wax may change its colour and consistency, which may prevent it from setting. Also, the smell of pure Essential Oil in the hot wax may be overpowering as the heat of the wax can cause the oil to evaporate very quickly, so ensure that the room is well ventilated and that you let the wax cool slightly before adding the oil.

Candlelight is the next best thing to an open fire. Warming and flattering to the eye, candles are the ideal way to create an atmosphere at a romantic dinner for two, or even for a swinging party that stretches into the early hours of the morning. Hand-made candles make great gifts, and what better way to brighten up someone's life?

Many pre-scented candles are available, but try and buy those with natural rather than synthetic fragrances.

Wood fire

There is nothing more romantic that sitting in front of a real fire, the warmth allowing your body to relax and your mind to wander. Put a maximum of 12 drops of Essential Oil on three pieces of wood about 15 minutes prior to burning to allow the fragrance of the Essential Oil to fill the room as the wood is warmed and eventually burned.

To create a clean, stimulating aroma try using Eucalyptus, Fennel, Juniperberry, Niaouli, Rosewood or Scots Pine. For a relaxing atmosphere you may wish to use Bergamot, Chamomile, Frankincense, Lavender, Myrrh, Orange or Petitgrain. If you are looking for a romantic ambience, use Patchouli, Sandalwood or Ylang Ylang.

Pot-pourri

A pot-pourri is one of the easiest ways to bring your house to life. Not only can you create a fragrance for any room, but you also have the visual stimulation of varied shapes and colours mixed together to create an interesting feature. The reputation of pot-pourri has been harmed by the wide availability of bags of very inexpensive flower-heads and leaves treated with cheap synthetic fragrances, while good-quality pot-pourri tends to be quite expensive. So why not try making your own?

Collect flower-heads, herbs, grasses and seed pods and dry them. Natural dyes can be introduced before drying, either by spraying the pot-pourri ingredients lightly with a vegetable-based dye or soaking them in a bowl of dye. You could even make your own dyes: beetroot gives a deep, dark red colour, and spinach can add a deep green colour. Allow about six weeks for your pot-pourri to dry, leaving it in a warm but well-ventilated place.

The pot-pourri can then be fragranced by placing it in a bag or airtight box and sprinkling it with a few drops of your favourite Essential Oil. Leave for a few hours before shaking the contents well; if a stronger fragrance is required, add more oil and leave for longer. Your pot-pourri will fragrance a room for up to six weeks; to revitalise it, just add more oil.

Flowers

There is nothing nicer than a vase of fresh-cut flowers in the house, but it is so disappointing when they have no fragrance. This can easily be rectified by adding an Essential Oil to the water or by dipping the stem of each flower into a blend of oil before arranging then in the vase. This allows the flower to absorb the oil up the stem and into the head, giving an attractive fragrance that will fool even the smartest of insects!

For dried flower arrangements, put a few drops of oil either on the flower-heads or on to the base. You could also apply a light mist of concentrated room spray over the arrangement.

Vacuuming

To keep your home clean and smelling fresh, place a few drops of Essential Oil on a ball of cotton-wool and place it in your vacuum-cleaner bag, if possible near the exit filter. To change or refresh the fragrance, just use a new cotton-wool ball as required.

Room sprays

See page 29.

Insect repellents

During the warm summer months our homes are invaded by hundreds of insects who smell the often sweet aroma within. An empty jam jar may attract a multitude of insects, but they will not stop there; they go back for reinforcements and before long you are sharing your home with a whole host of small creatures both with and without wings: silver fish on a tiled floor, ants around a doorway, fleas in our carpets and furniture, bees, wasps and moths. This is a problem not only at home but also on holiday, with sometimes the added aggravation of mosquitoes.

There are several Essential Oils that act as insect repellents: Cedarwood, Citronella, Eucalyptus, Juniperberry, Lemongrass, Litsea Cubeba and Tea Tree. These can be used as room sprays, in a room burner or applied in a soapy water solution to areas outside the home where insects enter. The smell will deter their entry, but unfortunately will not show the way out to those already in your home, so oils are best used as a preventative measure.

Aromatherapy in the bedroom and bathroom

We spend on average 121 days a year in our bed. Sleep is one thing we cannot do without: it allows our body to relax and repair itself and our minds to rest, and lets us start each day refreshed. However, for many this is not the case. Insomnia is a growing problem and many people can only dream of a good night's sleep.

Many Essential Oils have sedative properties and can help you drift off into a natural sleep without leaving you lethargic or heavy-eyed in the morning. They are also non-addictive, unlike some similar treatments in conventional medication. It is, of course, also important to have a firm but comfortable bed that supports your posture while also allowing you to relax. Many back problems are caused or aggravated by a poor-quality or old mattress.

There are several ways to use Essential Oils in the bedroom. A few drops of Essential Oil can be placed on a small cloth and put in the tumble dryer for the final 5 minutes when you dry your sheets. Put a few drops on a tissue and leave it next to your pillow so that you can inhale the aroma during the night.

We sweat on average about half a litre of fluid each night, and in warm conditions our beds can become a breeding ground for bacteria and bed mites. Cedarwood, a natural insecticide and also a sedative oil, would be ideal to put in a room spray for use once a month to keep your bed fresh. If you wish to rid your bed of mites it is always best to vacuum the mattress before spraying and spray every other day for four treatments, as it can be several days before the young eggs hatch. Remember to avoid spraying over polished, laminated or plastic surfaces, and always keep the spray clear of electrical appliances.

Aromatherapy bags

Probably the most common type of Aromatherapy bag is that filled with dried lavender heads, often used to freshen clothes in a wardrobe or drawer. This is quickly and easily made by using two squares of fabric sewn together to form a pouch, and it can either be filled with a natural herb or flower, a synthetic filler or a natural pulse, which can absorb an Essential Oil and allow it to evaporate gently over time. To keep moths out of your wardrobes and cupboards try using Citronella, Lavender and Rosemary. To relax and enjoy a good night's sleep tie a bag to your bedpost with a few drops of Lavender, Marjoram, Neroli or Petitgrain, while Frankincense has been known to ward off nightmares.

Aromatherapy bags can also be hung in the car to eliminate unpleasant odours; use Bergamot, Lemon or Litsea Cubeba. Peppermint is particularly good, as it is said to relieve travel sickness. *Do not use relaxing oils while driving.*

Toilet, bath and sink

To give your bathroom a deep clean without using chemicals that may harm the environment, while also leaving a pleasant clean smell and the assurance of a germ-free zone try using Grapefruit, Lemon, Lemongrass, Niaouli, Palmarosa, Rosewood, Scots Pine or Tea Tree. These all have either bactericide or disinfectant properties.

Tea Tree oil has excellent antiseptic qualities and has been known to kill harmful bacteria even diluted down to one part in a hundred, and when mixed with Scots Pine it is the ultimate natural bug-buster.

Use any or a combination of the oils above in the final rinse water when you wash surfaces in the bathroom - a couple of drops will not only kill germs but also leave a beautiful fragrance. You can also put a couple of drops of the oils on the cardboard tube inside the toilet roll. The aroma will gradually be released into the atmosphere and the cleansing molecules will leave the area clean and fragrant.

Aromatherapy in the kitchen

Essential Oils can be used in a room burner either to simulate or suppress hunger. The citrus oils have a great effect on the appetite as they stimulate the salivary glands and produce digestive acid in the stomach ready to break down the forthcoming food. Food seems to taste far nicer when we are hungry, and this could be a compensation if your culinary skills leave something to be desired! Essential Oils are burned in some restaurants to make people feel hungry, and since our eyes are usually bigger than our stomachs we may order more food than we would normally do! Supermarkets have been known to reproduce the smell of baking bread to encourage people to buy more because they feel hungry.

The reverse can be said of Fennel, Patchouli and Rosemary, which appear to suppress the appetite. These oils are particularly useful if you are on a weight-reducing diet or have recently given up smoking and want to prevent between-meal snacking.

Adding oils to washing-up liquid

You may wish to add an Essential Oil to your washing-up liquid to help with the removal of grease, bacteria or just for the pleasant fragrance. A few drops of either Bergamot; Lavender; Lime or Orange added to the washing-up water will change the way you wash up and will still be kind to your hands. You can use the same mixture to wipe clean your refrigerator, microwave or other kitchen appliance.

Sterilising dishes and cutlery

Bacteria breed faster in the kitchen and bathroom than anywhere else in the home, and the kitchen is a prime site for cross-contamination between raw and cooked food. It is easy to sterilise your dishes and cutlery by filling a bowl with hot water, adding a few drops of either Scots Pine or Tea Tree and rinsing the items, then drying them and returning them to the cupboards.

Kitchen surfaces, floors and boards

These areas are particularly prone to the spread of germs. Eucalyptus, Lavender, Lemon, Palmarosa and Tea Tree are all oils that can be used neat. Add them to hot water either with or without your detergent and you can be sure that your floors will not only look good but will provide protection for even the smallest members of the family.

For your work surfaces, add a few drops to water or apply directly on a cloth. Always remember that pure Essential Oils are very powerful and you only need a very small amount to do the job without leaving too much of an aroma. This also makes it an economical way to keep your home not just clean but *really* clean! Never use Essential Oils on polished or treated wooden surfaces without first testing their effect.

Kitchen smells

The kitchen is not always a place where nice smells are encountered, and Essential Oils can help here too, masking the stale smell of boiled cabbage, the powerful smell of a spicy take-away, damp coats, muddy boots and a bin full of rubbish, as well as their cleansing properties in a warm, moisture-filled environment where microscopic fat deposits make the perfect breeding ground for bacteria and nasty smells. It is easy to eliminate kitchen smells using Eucalyptus, Lavender, Lemon, Lemongrass, Lime or Litsea Cubeba. Use a room burner or pot-pourri, or hang dried flowers or herbs with a few drops of Essential Oil to keep that everyday fresh smell.

Laundry

Invigorating
Bergamot, Lemon, Litsea Cubeba, Petitgrain, Rosemary

Relaxing
Chamomile, Geranium, Lavender, Marjoram, Myrrh

Floral
Geranium, Jasmine, Lavender, Rose

Sensual
Myrrh, Patchouli, Sandalwood, Ylang Ylang

Chapter 8

Aromatherapy and animals

*F*or centuries Essential Oils have been used on humans to treat minor aliments, but recently more and more pet owners are bringing this more holistic approach to their animals. As explained earlier in this book, each Essential Oil has its own properties when used as a therapeutic remedy. The pain-killing action of Lavender and Marjoram, the relief of respiratory symptoms with Eucalyptus and Lemon, and the anti-arthritic effect of Juniperberry, Sandalwood and Scots Pine can have similar effects on animals.

Because of the diversity of pets and their many different bodily systems, animal Aromatherapy has become a very specialist field and is primarily controlled by veterinary surgeons who specialise in alternative therapies. However, the wide range of Essential Oils available can be used on most of our pets and there are now several good books that deal with this subject.

Just as with treating ourselves, there are two main ways to treat your pets: by inhalation or by massage with a blend of Essential Oils.

Inhalation

Inhalation can have some dramatic effects on animals, and many people who have been using Essential Oils for their own benefit have noticed marked effects of the behaviour of their animals. By using a room burner in your home as previously explained, the Essential Oil is allowed to evaporate into the air and can be breathed in by all the occupants of the house. However, beware of using too much Essential Oil, especially around cadged birds, as they have very small lungs and may find some oils too powerful. The same Essential Oils used in the room burner for humans can be used for many animals:

Lavender to calm and soothe, the citrus oils to stimulate and energise, and the herbal oils to aid with respiration and promote a healthy environment.

The other benefit of using a room burner is the pleasant aroma that will mask any unpleasant smells caused by animals. In addition, Essential Oils like Citronella and Lemongrass provide some protection against fleas and mites in the home as they are both natural insecticides. A spray can be made using Essential Oils and water to treat pet bedding and your home. As always, use Essential Oils with caution and always avoid polished surfaces.

Massage

Massage is one of the most commonly used methods of Aromatherapy for animals and can bring great relief to both animal and owner. It is well-known that pets have a great therapeutic affect on their owners, and the action of stroking an animal can lower your blood pressure and slow your heart rate. For the animal it allows muscle and soft tissue to be manipulated and stretched, bringing great relief to tired and aching limbs.

Neat Essential Oil should never be applied directly to the skin as it may cause a reaction or skin irritation. The structure of the skin will vary from breed to breed and even from animal to animal, so it is difficult to be specific about the strength of blends of Essential Oils to use, but as a general guide use 1 drop of Essential Oil to 10ml of a carrier oil for an animal the size of a small dog. Always skin-test your blend before applying it in any quantity, usually under the 'armpit' area or inner thigh where there is less fur. Leave it for a few minutes to see if there is any skin reaction or irritation before commencing the massage. In general 3 or 4 minutes of massage is sufficient to introduce the Essential Oil into the animal's system, and normally the treatment should be carried out twice a day for approximately five days.

Always remember that Aromatherapy is a complementary therapy and is not a substitute for veterinary care. There are many advantages to using Essential Oils on your animals; they are pleasant to use for both owner and pet, and are readily available. When buying oils for your animal ensure that they are pure

Essential Oils and not synthetically manufactured varieties, which do not have the same therapeutic qualities and can cause reactions on the skin of your animal, which in many cases can be more sensitive than your own.

Conditions and recommended treatments

The following dilution quantities are for the size of a small dog.

Abscess
Clean area around the abscess with 100 ml warm water containing 1 drop Lavender Essential Oil. After cleaning apply 1 drop Tea Tree Essential Oil to the abscess.

Aggression
Use a blend of 2 drops Sandalwood and 2 drops Ylang Ylang Essential Oil in 50 ml carrier and use as under 'Massage' above, or use either Essential Oil in a room burner.

Arthritis
See Rheumatism.

Bad breath
Blend 1 drop Lavender and 1 drop Myrrh Essential Oil with 5 ml carrier oil and add to the animal's food. Repeat weekly to keep bad breath at bay.

Cyst
Apply 1 drop neat Lavender or Tea Tree Essential Oil to the affected area.

Ear infection
Remove any discharge then massage around the area using 1 drop Tea Tree, 1 drop Lavender and 1 drop Chamomile Essential Oil in 5 ml carrier oil. Repeat daily until symptoms subside.

Fleas
An effective anti-flea recipe is a blend of 1 drop Cedarwood, 1 drop Lavender and 1 drop Citronella, applied to the outer side of an absorbent collar.

Minor burns, blisters, bites and cuts
Treat as for humans, using cold water to reduce the swelling and reduce the heat of the skin in the affected area. Apply neat Lavender Essential Oil as soon as possible, but do not cover the area.

Nervousness and hyperactivity
Blend 2 drops Chamomile, 3 drops Lavender and 1 drop Marjoram Essential Oil with 50 ml carrier oil and massage 5 ml of the blend twice daily for three days, then as required.

Respiratory problems
To bring relief, place a warm compress of Eucalyptus or Niaouli Essential Oil (2 drops to 1 pint warm water) on the back and chest. Alternatively use a room burner. Repeat twice daily.

For smaller animals use Eucalyptus, Peppermint or Tea Tree Essential Oils, either on the base of the neck or a few drops of either Essential Oil in hot soapy water to wash out cages/hutches.

Rheumatism/arthritis blend
Apply 2 drops Ginger, 1 drop Rosemary and 3 drops Chamomile Essential Oil to 25 ml carrier oil. Massage into the affected area, working the oil through the fur into the skin surrounding the affected joints.

Skin problems
Blend 5 drops Lavender and 5 drops Chamomile Essential Oil with 100 ml Evening Primrose Blend and apply over the affected area twice daily.

Travel sickness
Blend 1 drop Fennel, 1 drop Peppermint and 1 drop Chamomile with 25 ml Evening Primrose Carrier. Massage approximately 5 ml of the blend into the chest and back 30 minutes before travel.

Chapter 9

Aromatherapy and pregnancy

*F*rom the moment of conception everything eaten, drunk or applied to the skin of the pregnant mother is filtered through to the unborn child. *For this reason it is recommended that Essential Oils should NOT be used in physical applications during the first four months of pregnancy.* After that period the following Essential Oils may be used *in half dilution*: Chamomile, Frankincense, Lavender, Lime, Mandarin, Palmarosa, Petitgrain, Tea Tree and Neroli blend.

The Essential Oils may be used in a room burner; however, as with many things during pregnancy, your tastes will change and it is very much a case of trial and error in choosing the oils to suit your mood. Always take into account the general precautions (see Chapter 10).

Likisma's range of pre-blended Aromatherapy shampoos, conditioners, shower gels, bath soaks, and hand and foot treatments are perfectly safe to use during pregnancy. Bearing in mind again that the change in hormonal balance may affect skin sensitivity, it would be wise to do a patch test on the inner arm before use.

Antenatal care after four months

Backache
With the increasing weight of the baby, many women experience low back-ache during the later stages of pregnancy. Resting with the legs and feet raised will help to alleviate pain, as will gentle exercise such as yoga. *Gentle* massage will also be beneficial either with a carrier oil alone or a Neroli blend (2% or less) or perhaps a blend of 1-2 drops of Lavender to 10 ml of carrier oil. It may be necessary to

massage with the expectant mother laying on her side or in a sitting position, whichever is most comfortable for both parties.

Constipation
To help avoid constipation, drink plenty of plain bottled or filtered water - up to 2 litres a day. Combined with a healthy diet full of fresh vegetables and fruit, this will help to dispel unwanted toxins. Broccoli and cabbage are particularly good natural laxatives, as are prunes and figs.

Try a *very gentle* massage with a carrier oil in a clockwise direction over the abdomen starting by the right groin, up to the rib-cage, then across and down the left-hand side to the groin; repeat several times. This will help to activate bowel movement.

Cramp
Leg cramps in pregnancy are fairly common in the later months and soaking the feet in a bowl of warm water with 1 drop of Lavender and 1 drop of Chamomile will be both calming and soothing. In cases of calcium deficiency a calcium supplement may be prescribed.

Nausea
In most cases sickness subsides by the fourth month; 2-3 drops of either Ginger, Peppermint or Spearmint Essential Oil in a room burner might help.

Stretch marks
It is a good idea to massage the abdomen *gently* from the start with just a carrier oil. Grapeseed with added Wheatgerm is a particularly good source of vitamin E, A and B. The Wheatgerm will prolong the 'shelf life' of the carrier as well as helping to regenerate tissues and skin elasticity, making it the best oil to use for scar tissue and stretch marks (see page 33).

After five months Neroli blend, a good cocoa butter cream or a Lavender blend at half dilution lightly massaged on to the abdomen would be particularly soothing for both the mother-to-be and her baby.

Swollen ankles and feet

Again this is quite a common symptom of pregnancy (oedema) and is best dealt with by taking time out each day for leg rest. Lie down and place the feet and ankles on a pillow, keeping them higher than the heart for at least 20 minutes. This will help to drain excess fluid away from the ankles. A cold compress with Lavender or Chamomile may also be of benefit.

During labour

Back massage during labour and delivery is now widely accepted and encouraged. A Rose or Jasmine blend will not only aid contractions and relieve pain but will also produce a beautiful and pleasing aroma in the delivery room. Both of these Essential Oils are described as valuable uterine tonics.

To help relax everyone in the delivery room an alternative would be to put 2-3 drops of Lavender Essential Oil in a room burner or vaporiser, which will also help to cleanse the air.

Post-natal care

Personal hygiene is important at all times but even more so directly after childbirth. Taking regular baths (twice a day) for the first 10 days with Lavender and/or Chamomile will not only soothe bruised and delicate areas but will aid healing and fight infection. If you are breast-feeding use in half dilution.

Breast-feeding

It is again important to mention here that whatever the nursing mother uses on her skin (in however minute a quantity) will be absorbed and transmitted through her milk to the baby. With this in mind it is still recommended that the suggested Essential Oils are used in half dilution for physical application until such time as the baby is weaned. Chamomile and Lavender would still be first choice.

Cracked and sore nipples are a common problem when breast-feeding. Whether the hospital recommends the use of a cream or spray, or you massage with carrier oils, do make sure that all traces are removed before the baby feeds from the nipple.

Post-natal depression

This, or indeed any type of depression, can be relieved with the use of certain Essential Oils. It is very much personal taste, but the more uplifting are the citrus aromas of Bergamot, Grapefruit and Mandarin, while the balancing properties of Clary Sage, Geranium, Neroli and Rose are certainly to be considered. Use in the bath, room burner and massage; if you are breast-feeding, use the room burner method only and consult your doctor or midwife. *If at all in doubt, take professional advice.*

Chapter 10

General precautions

*U*nfortunately there are at present no regulations regarding Essential Oils. There are proposals currently at the European Union to establish a registration system for all complementary therapist practitioners and suppliers, but this will take some time to be enacted, if ever!

You will find many chemists, drug stores, specialist shops and other retail outlets now selling Essential Oils and other Aromatherapy goods. There are also several mail order companies offering Essential Oils to the public. We cannot, of course, comment on the quality or purity of all the products on offer. You must try to make sure that wherever you purchase your oils they are consistent with the descriptions given in the previous chapter and actually work in the way they are supposed to. (See 'Quality of oils' in Chapter 1.)

Essential Oils are a natural product, which, if used correctly, can be safer than using pharmacological preparations because they have a gentler effect on the human system with far less, if any, side-effects. However, in the detailed list of oils on the previous pages there were some precautions attached to most of them. Apart from these specific precautions there are some general points about Essential Oils that need to be borne in mind when they are used.

1   With any **major condition**, for example high blood pressure, arthritis, measles, etc, **always consult your GP** before attempting treatment with Aromatherapy. Although there are many medical practitioners who still do not believe in the benefits of Aromatherapy or other complementary therapies it is always wise to seek your doctor's advice about using Essential Oils.

2   If you are already **taking prescribed medications** for any condition, again consult your doctor or a qualified

Aromatherapist before using Essential Oils. There is a possibility that the chemical constituents in all Essential Oils will interact with the chemicals in the prescribed medication, which at best may neutralise each other and at worst create more problems.

Medication and all other chemical preparations that you buy 'over the counter', for example aspirin, Panadol, Friar's Balsam; calamine lotion, etc, will usually be safe to use at the same time as using Essential Oils. If you do feel a reaction to using oils then immediately stop using them, drink plenty of water, and massage the body with the carrier oil alone. If the reaction persists, consult your doctor.

3   Essential Oils will not normally react negatively to **naturopathic or homoeopathic remedies**. Treat as medication and follow your therapist's directions.

4   Never exceed the **maximum dosage** recommended. Most Aromatherapists agree that this is a 2-3% dilution, which can be measured as 1 drop of Essential Oil to every 2 millilitres or grams of base (for sensitive skin see precaution 13). In baths this dilution will be much less (we recommend a maximum of 6 drops of Essential Oils). In general always work on the principle of the less the better. A minimum dosage would be 1 drop of Essential Oil to every 5 millilitres or grams of base. *Use half quantity of Essential Oils for facial use.*

5   Do not use one oil, or blend of oils, consistently over a long period of time (ie every day for three or more weeks). **Always vary the oils** that you use to prevent the body becoming immune to their effects and to avoid the possibility of a toxic build-up. You will see from the previous chapters that there are always alternative oils you can use for a particular condition.

6   **Never use** the following oils, as they have been demonstrated to be toxic and should only be used as directed by a qualified Aromatherapist, if at all:

ALMOND (BITTER) *Prunus amygdalis*
ANISEED *Pimpinella anisum*
BOLDO LEAF *Peumus boldus*
CALAMUS *Acorus calamus*
CAMPHOR (BROWN) *Cinnamomum camphora*
CAMPHOR (YELLOW) *Cinnamomum camphora*
CASSIA *Cinnamomum cassia*
CINNAMON BARK *Cinnamomum zeylanicum*
CLOVE BUD *Eugenia caryophyllata*
CLOVE LEAF *Eugenia caryophyllata*
CLOVE STEM *Eugenia caryophyllata*
COSTUS *Saussurea lappa*
ELECAMPANE *Inula helenium*
FENNEL (BITTER) *Foeniculum vulgare*
HORSERADISH *Cochlearia armoricia*
HYSSOP *Hyssopus officinalis*
JABORANDI LEAF *Pilocarpus jaborandi*
MUGWORT (ARMOISE) *Artemisia vulgaris*
MUSTARD *Brassica nigra*
ORIGANUM *Origanum vulgare*
ORIGANUM (SPANISH) *Thymus capitatus*
PENNYROYAL (EUROPEAN) *Mentha pulegium*
PENNYROYAL (AMERICAN) *Hedeoma pulegioides*
PINE (DWARF) *Pinus pumilio*
RUE *Ruta graveolens*
SAGE *Salvia officinalis*
SASSAFRAS *Sassafras albidum*
SASSAFRAS (BRAZIL) *Ocotea cymbarum*
SAVIN *Juniperus sabina*
SAVORY (SUMMER) *Satureia hortensis*
SAVORY (WINTER) *Satureia montana*
SOUTHERNWOOD *Artemisia abrotanum*
TANSY *Tanacetum vulgare*
THUJA (CEDARLEAF) *Thuja occidentalis*
THUJA PLICATA *Thuja plicata*
WINTERGREEN *Gaultheria procumbens*
WORMSEED *Chenopodium anthelminticum*
WORMWOOD *Artemisia absinthium*

This list was first prepared for the International Federation of Aromatherapists and is one we would endorse.

7   **Babies, infants and children** require a different dosage from adults, and some oils are not suitable for use with babies and infants at all. There is a great deal of controversy around this issue amongst Aromatherapists and the range of opinions can run from the use of any oil for any age at one extreme to the non-use of any oil for a child at the other extreme. Make sure your oils have child-proof caps.

Our view is that there are some restrictions to the use of Essential Oils with non-adults. We would suggest:

Babies (birth-4 years): We recommend that you only use Lavender and Chamomile for this age group. Use in minute dosages (1 drop to every 7 or 8 ml base) for direct application methods. When using in the bath always blend the Essential Oil with 10 ml of Sweet Almond carrier oil first before adding to the bath (or use a bath carrier).

Infants (4-7 years): Chamomile and Lavender can be used in half dosages at this age, ie 1 drop to every 4 ml. The following oils can be used at quarter strength (try skin test first - 1 drop to 8 ml carrier oil) Cedarwood, Mandarin, Myrtle, Palmarosa, Rose, Spearmint, Tangerine and Tea Tree.

Children (7-12 years): All oils listed in the alphabetical list in Chapter 6 can be used. Use in half the adult dosage and monitor reactions carefully.

It is important to understand that these recommendations are precautionary. All children, as with all adults, will have different levels of sensitivity to different oils, so take your cue from your child - you know them better than anyone else!

8   Do not use the following oils before going out into **strong sunshine** or using **sunbeds:** Bergamot; Citronella; Grapefruit; Lemon; Lime; Orange; Mandarin; Tangerine. They react to ultraviolet light making skin more sensitive.

9   With **high blood pressure** avoid Rosemary.

10   In **Epilepsy** avoid Basil, Eucalyptus and Fennel. Use Rosemary
     in minimum dosage only.

11   If **diabetic** avoid Eucalyptus, Geranium and Lemon.

12   We recommend Essential Oils should not be used in physical
     applications in the first 4 months of **pregnancy**. After such time
     we recommend the following in half dilution: Chamomile,
     Frankincense, Lavender, Lime, Mandarin, Palmarosa,
     Petitgrain, Tea Tree and Neroli blend.

13   For **sensitive skin** always try a skin test before using any
     Essential Oil. Dilute 2 drops of the Essential Oil with 5 ml of
     carrier oil and massage into the inner/upper arm. If there is no
     reaction within 5-10 minutes you should be safe to use the oil.
     There are several oils that could irritate sensitive skin: Basil;
     Bergamot; Black Pepper; Citronella; Coriander; Fennel;
     Ginger; Grapefruit; Lemon; Lemongrass; Lime; Litsea Cubeba;
     Orange; Peppermint; Scots Pine; Tea Tree; Ylang Ylang.

14   **Essential Oils must *never* be used on the eyes.** If any oil comes
     into contact with your eyes, flush it out with Sweet Almond
     carrier oil. Water will only make the situation worse. Usually
     the oil will only make your eyes sting a little for a while. If pain
     persists consult your doctor.

15   **NEVER USE ESSENTIAL OILS INTERNALLY.** This again is
     an area of controversy within Aromatherapy. Some
     Aromatherapists will say that taking some oils orally, in minute
     dosage and diluted in something else, is acceptable. Others will
     say that using oils in the mouth for dental problems or as a
     mouthwash is acceptable but would not recommend ingestion.
     Some, like ourselves, do not favour any oral or ingestive use of
     oils. A recent statement by the Aromatherapy Trade Council,
     an organisation for companies and organisations trading in
     Aromatherapy products in the UK who conform to a set of
     standards set down by the ATC, backs up this view:
        'The ATC feels that unless a substance is licensed by the

Medicines Control Agency as a medical product it should not be taken orally.' (quoted in *Journal of Alternative & Complementary Medicine*, Vol 13, No 6, p 6)

There is evidence that ingested oils are neither effective nor safe. The terpenes in them are irritating to the sensitive membranes in the digestive tract and can cause damage. The stomach is a very hostile place to the delicate balance of chemicals in Essential Oils and rapidly destroys any use the oils might have been. **IF YOU OR YOUR CHILD ACCIDENTALLY SWALLOWS** oils consult your doctor immediately. Always buy oils in bottles with child-resistant caps.

Please do not be put off by these precautions! You will see that most are exactly that - a precaution - and if treated sensibly and with respect everyone can gain a great deal of benefit and pleasure from the use of Essential Oils. Try them and see!

Further reading

Arnould-Taylor, W. E. *A Textbook of Holistic Aromatherapy* (Stanley Thornes Ltd)
  The Principles & Practice of Physical Therapy (Stanley Thornes Ltd)
Britt, Jennifer *Peppermint* (Silver Link Publishing Ltd)
Chambers, Philip (ITEC Dip) *The Very Essence of Massage* (Likisma Presentations Limited)
Davis, Patricia *Aromatherapy: an A-Z* (C. W. Daniel Co Ltd)
Del Gaudio Mak, Marion *Aroma Therapy, Simply for You* (Amberwood Ltd)
Drury, Susan *Tea Tree Oil* (C. W. Daniel Co Ltd)
Kusmirek, Jan (Ed) *Aromatherapy for the Family* (Institute of Classical Aromatherapy; Wigmore Publications Ltd)
Lavabre, Marcel F. *Aromatherapy Workbook* (Healing Arts Press)
Maxwell-Hudson, Clare, and others *The Book of Massage* (Ebury Press)
  The Complete Book of Massage (Dorling Kindersley)
Mitchell, Stewart *Massage, A practical introduction* (Element)
Price, Shirley *Practical Aromatherapy* (Thorsons)
Ryman, Daniele *Aromatherapy* (Piatkus)
Sellar, Wanda *The Directory of Essential Oils* (C. W. Daniel Co Ltd)
Smith, Dr Tony (Ed) *MacMillan Guide to Family Health* (MacMillan Ltd)
Tisserand, Maggie *Aromatherapy for Lovers* (Thorsons)
  Aromatherapy for Women (Thorsons)
Tisserand, Robert *The Art of Aromatherapy* (C. W. Daniel Co Ltd)
Westwood, Christine *Aromatherapy* (Amberwood Ltd)
  Aromatherapy, Stress Management (Amberwood Ltd)
  Aromatherapy (Element)
  Holistic Aromatherapy (Thorsons)
Worwood, Valerie Ann *The Fragrant Pharmacy* (Bantam Books)